Get Through

Nuclear Medicine for the FRCR and MRCP

Get Through

Nuclear Medicine for the FRCR and MRCP

John Frank
MSc FRCP FRCR
Consultant in Nuclear Medicine and Radiology
Charing Cross Hospital
London

Thomas Nunan
MSc MD FRCP FRCR
Consultant Physician
Guy's and St Thomas' Hospitals NHS Trust
London

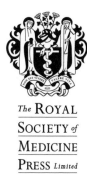

The ROYAL
SOCIETY of
MEDICINE
PRESS Limited

© 2004 Royal Society of Medicine Press Ltd

Published by the Royal Society of Medicine Press Ltd
1 Wimpole Street, London W1G 0AE, UK
Tel: +44 (0)20 7290 2921
Fax: +44 (0)20 7290 2929
E-mail: publishing@rsm.ac.uk
Website: www.rsmpress.co.uk

British Library Cataloguing in Publication Data
A catalogue record for this book is available from the British Library

ISBN 1-85315-550-0

Distribution in Europe and Rest of World:
Marston Book Services Ltd
PO Box 269
Abingdon
Oxon OX14 4YN, UK
Tel: +44 (0)1235 465500
Fax: +44 (0)1235 465555

Distribution in the USA and Canada:
Royal Society of Medicine Press Ltd
c/o Jamco Distribution Inc
1401 Lakeway Drive
Lewisville, TX 75057, USA
Tel: +1 800 538 1287
Fax: +1 972 353 1303
E-mail: jamco@majors.com

Distribution in Australia and New Zealand:
Elsevier Australia
30–52 Smidmore Street
Marrickville, NSW 2204
Australia
Tel: +612 9517 8999
Fax: +612 9517 2249
E-mail: service@elsevier.com.au

Phototypeset by Phoenix Photosetting, Chatham, Kent
Printed by Bell & Bain Ltd, Glasgow

Contents

Foreword

Nuclear medicine in the UK is a small specialty with a very broad range of applications which include the use of unsealed radiation sources for therapy and tracer techniques for pathophysiological investigation. In this book, the authors have concentrated entirely on the radionuclide imaging component of nuclear medicine, which is the most relevant area for postgraduate training in radiology and clinical medicine.

The thought processes involved in medical imaging diagnosis remain elusive and intriguing. In recent years much has been said and written about 'pattern recognition' and there is no doubt that this approach makes an important contribution to image interpretation. However, it is equally certain that there is more to it than that. We need also to understand the mechanisms by which disease alters anatomy and physiology to produce changes in the diagnostic image, and further we need to understand the physical principles of image production. The teaching cases which make up this book are presented with questions which seek out this underlying knowledge, as well as the ability to perceive the abnormal features in the images. Specific teaching points are highlighted for each case and, where appropriate, the educational value is further enhanced by the inclusion of correlative imaging.

This book is not a substitute for the systematic teaching and study of radionuclide imaging, but it does cover a very broad range of different clinical applications in nuclear imaging techniques. As such it offers an effective test of knowledge and interpretative ability across the spectrum of clinical radionuclide imaging which not only mimics the viva voce component of the postgraduate examinations, but also reflects real-life diagnostic problems.

In the UK the specialties of nuclear medicine and radiology are becoming ever more closely associated, and it is a particular pleasure for me that this book – which is aimed at trainees in both disciplines – has been co-authored by a radiologist and a nuclear physician.

Professor Philip Robinson
Professor of Imaging
St James's Hospital
Leeds

Preface

This book has been written to give trainee radiologists and physicians exposure to a wide range of conditions commonly investigated using Nuclear Medicine techniques. It is presented in a question and answer format which a candidate might expect to encounter in their higher professional examinations.

Both static and dynamic studies are included in a series of cases, with correlative imaging where appropriate. Teaching points are included. Whilst following the new FRCR syllabus, where Nuclear Medicine may constitute as much as 20%, the cases are presented in a random order, as in an exam.

Nuclear Medicine has advanced out of all recognition in the past decade; a glance at the contents page of any of the Nuclear Medicine journals will pinpoint the main cause – PET, and the even more exciting combined PET/CT scanners, which firmly link nuclear medicine to cross-sectional imaging. However, there are many other Nuclear Medicine investigations and they play a complementary role to other forms of imaging. This is reflected in such higher exams as the FRCR and the MRCP.

Following the cases, a short section covers such important topics as regulatory issues and how to continue in Nuclear Medicine after the FRCR and MRCP.

John and Tom

Acknowledgements

The images used in this book have been collected by us over the years from all the hospitals we have worked in, but we would like to acknowledge our colleagues who have provided images, and in particular Dr Adam Mitchell for MRI images of pars defects.

We would also like to thank Amersham plc for permission to use the composite DAT image demonstrating the severity of Parkinson's disease.

The authors would especially like to thank their wives and families for help and support.

Cases

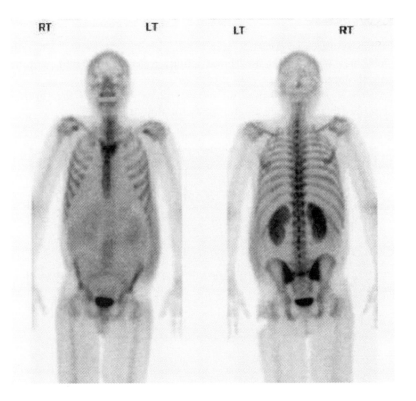

This bone scan shows an interesting incidental finding.

1. What is it?
2. What imaging would you do next?

ANSWERS

1. Diffusely increased uptake is clearly seen within the abdomen. This is due to ascites and the increased bone activity reflects the altered peritoneal metabolism.
2. Ascites is easily confirmed on ultrasound, which shows the shrunken knobbly liver and large amount of ascitic fluid.

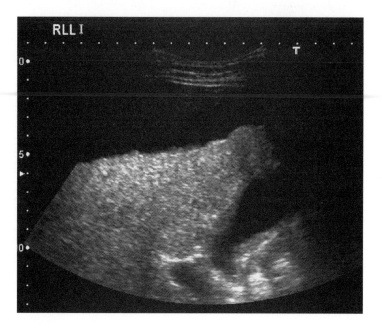

TEACHING POINT

- Although bone scans primarily show the skeleton, remember that bone agent will also appear in areas where there is damage to the blood–structure barrier, as here where there is an inflammatory reaction due to the ascites. Bone agent is also seen in other sites where there is an inflammatory reaction, e.g. in breast carcinomas. (A more exhaustive list is given on p 32.)

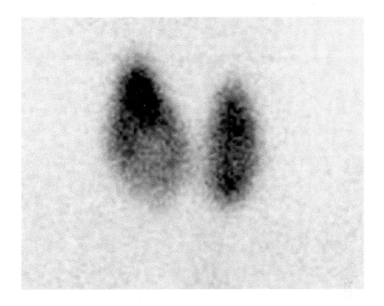

This patient presented with a lump in the lower part of the right side of the neck.

1. What does this image show?
2. What is the clinical role of this test in the evaluation of thyroid masses?
3. What other investigation would you perform?

ANSWERS

1. This is a ^{99m}Tc thyroid scan. It shows a cold nodule in the right lobe of the thyroid.
2. Isotope scanning is of value in cases where it is suspected that the nodule might be functioning since functioning nodules are very rarely malignant. Care must be taken with 'warm' nodules, since the incidence of malignancy is higher in these. Isotope scanning is also useful in establishing whether the gland has a single or multiple nodules.
3. Ultrasound of the solitary cold nodule is mandatory and will show whether the lesion is cystic or solid. Ultrasound can also establish whether the gland has a single or multiple nodules.

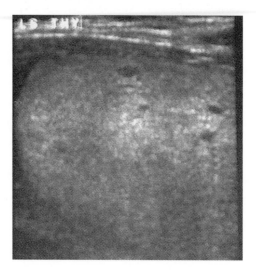

The above ultrasound shows that the nodule is solid. Solid cold nodules may have malignant foci and a fine needle aspiration (FNA) should be performed. The Thyroid Association Guideline (www.british-thyroid-association.org) states that ultrasound is of value to direct the FNA. Where any doubt about the pathology exists, the lobe should be removed. Cystic solitary nodules may be left and followed up with ultrasound, or aspirated.

TEACHING POINTS

- A careful history should be obtained, especially in cases of previous head and neck cancer, as the palpable lump may be a secondary deposit. In such cases, ultrasound and PET scanning are the investigations of choice.
- As the aim is to exclude malignancy in a euthyroid patient, imaging should only be performed if there are specific indications, and it should not delay a tissue diagnosis. The precise incidence of malignancy in thyroid nodules is debated. The difficulty is that there is a significant selection bias in series in which surgery is used as the diagnostic test. The figure used in practice is $\leq 10\%$ of thyroid nodules are malignant.

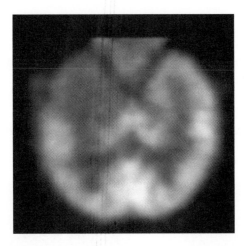

1. What tracer is this?
2. What does the scan show?
3. Suggest a clinical indication for this investigation.

ANSWERS

1. An ^{18}F-FDG PET brain scan in a patient with a glioma.
2. Diminished activity in the right frontal area.
3. The indication for the scan is two-fold: (i) to establish the grade of tumour in the primary work-up; and (ii) in follow-up to look for recurrent disease.

MRI will show the extent of disease, but will not demonstrate the metabolism within the tumour.

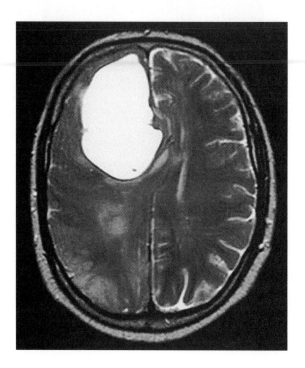

TEACHING POINTS

- The cause of the globally reduced uptake in the right temporal lobe will depend on the clinical circumstances: low-grade gliomas, post-radiotherapy changes or, in a non-tumour setting, epilepsy.
- High-grade gliomas take up FDG more avidly than normal cortex and low-grade tumours take up FDG less avidly than normal cortex. Thus, the PET scan can determine the grade of tumour. Prognosis is related to the grade.
- PET can also differentiate recurrence in high-grade tumours, but because of the reduced uptake in lower grade tumours, the detection of recurrence is less accurate.

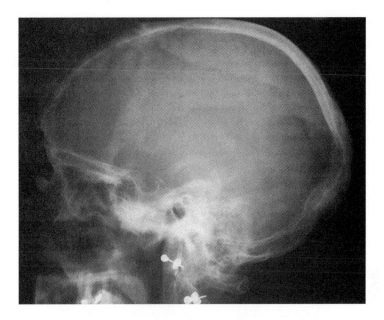

This elderly patient presented with diminished mobility and was found to have a raised alkaline phosphatase on routine testing. This is the skull X-ray.

1. What does it show?
2. What imaging would you do next?

ANSWERS

1. The lateral skull X-ray shows some porosis anteriorly and slight fuzziness of the outer table. This is typical of osteoporosis circumscripta, an early, aggressive and metabolically active form of Paget's disease of the skull.
2. A conventional bone scan will show the extent of the Paget's, which may be much greater than seen on X-ray.

The scan below shows the increased activity throughout the skull.

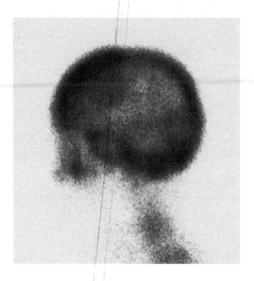

Paget's may affect any bone, and in long bones usually, but not always, starts at an articular surface. Below is an example of Paget's of a digit.

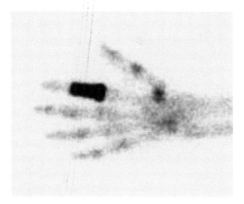

TEACHING POINT

- Paget's disease is often found by chance and is said to occur in 5% of the elderly. There is a <1% risk of the Paget's becoming malignant (osteo-sarcoma). Typically, it affects long bones from an articular surface along the shaft, and the bone appears enlarged on X-ray.

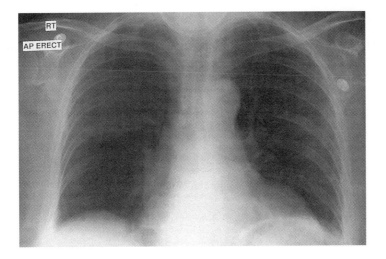

This patient recently had a total knee replacement and became dyspnoeic and hypoxic.

1. What does this image show?
2. What diagnoses would you consider?
3. What investigation would you do next?

ANSWERS

1. The chest X-ray is normal.
2. Possible diagnoses are pulmonary embolism (PE) or pneumothorax.
3. AV/Q lung scan. This uses ^{99m}Tc-MAA microspheres and ^{81m}Kr gas.

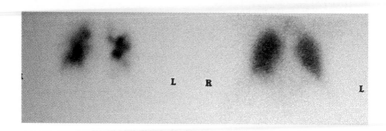

The scan above shows multiple perfusion defects in the perfusion image (left) which are not matched on the ventilation image (right), which is normal. This is diagnostic of multiple PEs.

TEACHING POINTS

- ^{81m}Kr ventilation images can be identified by seeing the gas in the trachea, as above.
- Whenever there is clinical suspicion of PE, a lung scan should be performed. There are PIOPED criteria for assessing the probability of PEs: high, intermediate, low and normal.
  - *High* is two large or four smaller perfusion defects, with normal ventilation and chest X-ray. Where defects are in both lungs, as above, the diagnosis is much more obvious.
  - *Intermediate* is classed as not falling into either *high* or *low* probabilities.
  - *Low* is one moderate mismatched defect with a normal chest X-ray; non-segmental perfusion defects; any perfusion defect with a sub-stantially larger chest X-ray abnormality; large or moderate matched defects in either one or both lungs.
- In all cases where a lung scan is performed, a recent chest X-ray must be available.
- Where there is a high clinical suspicion, treatment should be started straight away and not be delayed by waiting for a lung scan. The lung scan will be positive for up to 8 days after the PE. Obviously, a scan should be obtained as soon as possible after the event.
- In pneumothorax, the perfusion and ventilation scans are normal, but are smaller than on the unaffected side, due to the lung collapse.

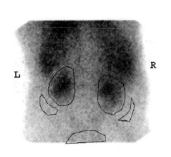

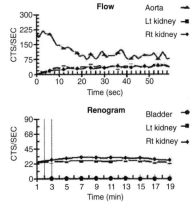

1. What is this investigation?
2. What does it show?

ANSWERS

1. A MAG3 dynamic renogram, labelled with ^{99m}Tc. The patient presented with renal failure and a high creatinine, and the ultrasound showed normal collecting systems. In this situation, it is not usually necessary to stress the kidneys with furosemide.
2. This scan is abnormal. It shows (left) the summed view with the regions of interest drawn around the kidneys, background, heart and bladder. The background activity is rather high. The computer then generates two sets of curves (right). The upper set shows the clearance through the heart and into the kidneys. There is symmetrical but diminished inflow of isotope into the kidneys. The lower graph shows the clearance of isotope and hardly any clearance is seen, although each kidney contributes roughly 50% of total renal function. The two parallel lines between 2 and 3 min are the conventional time when the relative function is calculated.

TEACHING POINTS

- In renal failure, there is usually very poor excretion and the renogram curves are flat, as here, but there is no evidence of obstruction.
- The higher the creatinine, the higher the background activity.
- MAG3 is filtered by the glomeruli and secreted into the renal space in the renal tubules. Thus, it has a better extraction fraction than the alternative tracer for renography – DTPA, which is only filtered. This makes MAG3 a superior imaging agent for renography, especially when there is impaired renal function.
- Delayed images may be helpful if there is a suspicion of outflow tract obstruction.
- Compare these curves to the normal dynamic renogram.

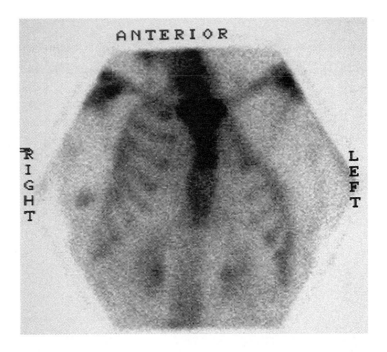

This is an anterior view of the thorax from a bone scan series.

1. What does it show?

ANSWER

1. Distortion of the left side of the thorax and a dorsal scoliosis convex to the left.

The distortion is due to a left-sided thoracoplasty, a procedure carried out many years ago for tuberculosis before effective antituberculous drugs were available. Such operations were common and patients are still occasionally seen who have had this procedure.

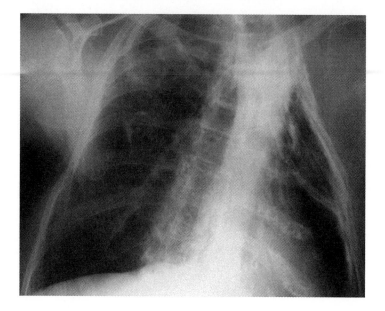

The left thoracoplasty and evidence of old tuberculosis are clearly seen on the X-ray above.

TEACHING POINTS

- Where there is distortion of the anatomy on the bone scan, think of previous surgery.
- Another therapeutic intervention that affects bone scans is radiotherapy, which causes a region of reduced uptake.
- Surgery, e.g. a sternal split, will cause increased uptake and it can take up to a year before the scan is normal again.
- In patients with pathology in a lower limb, e.g. old polio, increased uptake is often seen on the normal side, caused by increased weight bearing on the 'good' leg.

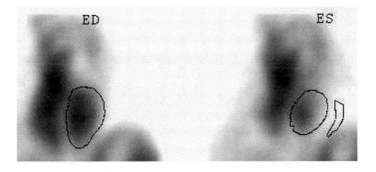

1. What are these images and what do they represent?
2. What radiopharmaceutical is used?
3. How is the test performed and why?

ANSWERS

1. Smoothed summed images showing the amount of activity within the left ventricle of the heart at end diastole (ED) and end systole (ES). They form part of a cardiac MUltiple Gated Acquisition study (MUGA).
2. The basis of this test is to label the patient's own red cells using an intra-venous injection of stannous chloride, which is cleared from the plasma and penetrates the red cells where it is reduced. This makes the red cells susceptible to ^{99m}Tc pertechnetate, a dose of which is then injected after 20 min. This labels the red cells *in vivo*.
3. The patient is then connected to an ECG monitor which feeds the signal to the gamma-camera. The camera acquires data during the R–R interval and builds up a series of frames during the study. These are then replayed as a ciné loop on the gamma-camera computer system, and thus the motion of the left ventricle wall can be assessed. The computer processing program will give the ejection fraction (EF), and create an image showing ED and ES superimposed.

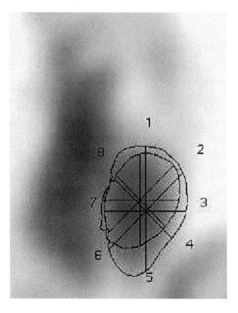

The test is used whenever a simple EF calculation is required, and mainly to monitor the results of cardiotoxic chemotherapy in malignancy.

TEACHING POINT

- The test is simple to perform and gives good reproducible results, hence its use in chemotherapy surveillance.

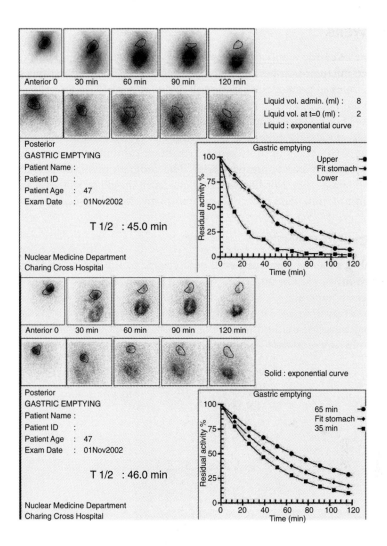

Anterior 0   30 min   60 min   90 min   120 min

Liquid vol. admin. (ml) :   8
Liquid vol. at t=0 (ml) :   2
Liquid : exponential curve

Posterior
GASTRIC EMPTYING
Patient Name :
Patient ID :
Patient Age : 47
Exam Date : 01Nov2002

T 1/2 : 45.0 min

Nuclear Medicine Department
Charing Cross Hospital

Gastric emptying
Upper
Fit stomach
Lower
Residual activity %
Time (min)

Anterior 0   30 min   60 min   90 min   120 min

Solid : exponential curve

Posterior
GASTRIC EMPTYING
Patient Name :
Patient ID :
Patient Age : 47
Exam Date : 01Nov2002

T 1/2 : 46.0 min

Nuclear Medicine Department
Charing Cross Hospital

Gastric emptying
65 min
Fit stomach
35 min
Residual activity %
Time (min)

This patient presented to the gastroenterology department complaining of severe reflux oesophagitis. He was an insulin-dependent diabetic.

1. What do these graphs show?
2. How are the graphs achieved?

ANSWERS

1. Rate of gastric emptying with solid and liquid components.
2. Two different isotopes are used. The solid meal, usually something bland like mashed potato, is labelled with a low dose of ^{99m}Tc-tin colloid, and the liquid component, usually orange juice, is labelled with a low dose of ^{111}In-DTPA. Dual acquisition allows the patient to consume solid and liquid at the same time, and then images are obtained at 30 min intervals over 2 h. Regions of interest are drawn around the stomach and time–activity curves are produced. The program gives the half-life for both phases. The half-life for liquid clearance should be <30 min and for solid <90 min. This study shows abnormally slow clearance of liquid.

TEACHING POINTS

- This test can be combined with oesophageal transit studies, and both are superior to barium studies in providing physiological information about rates of emptying.
- The normal variance is quite high and each department needs to establish a reproducible method of feeding and methodology. Nevertheless, useful physiological data is obtained.

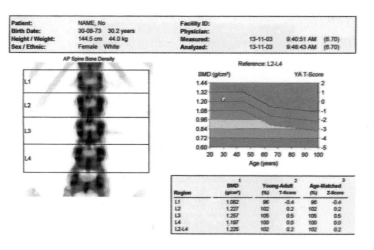

Patient:	NAME, No		Facility ID:			
Birth Date:	30-08-73	30.2 years	Physician:			
Height / Weight:	144.5 cm	44.0 kg	Measured:	13-11-03	9:40:51 AM	(6.70)
Sex / Ethnic:	Female	White	Analyzed:	13-11-03	9:48:43 AM	(6.70)

AP Spine Bone Density

Reference: L2-L4

Region	BMD¹ (g/cm²)	Young-Adult² (%)	T-Score	Age-Matched³ (%)	Z-Score
L1	1.082	96	-0.4	96	-0.4
L2	1.227	102	0.2	102	0.2
L3	1.257	105	0.5	105	0.5
L4	1.197	100	0.0	100	0.0
L2-L4	1.225	102	0.2	102	0.2

1. What is this scan?

ANSWER

1. A DXA scan, which is used to demonstrate bone density.

Typically, the lumbar spine is scanned from L1–4 and the pelvis. The results are expressed as g/cm^2, with reference to a database collected from normal age/sex matched cases. Where the patient has total hip replacements, the pelvis is not imaged.

Errors can arise when there is significant degenerative disease in the lumbar spine, or there is osteoporotic collapse. On a bone scan, osteoporotic collapse is typically shown as even plate-like increased uptake. Compare the image below with the case shown on p 104.

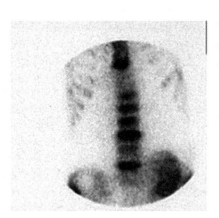 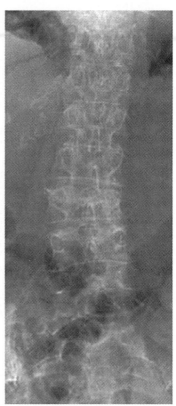

TEACHING POINT

- Before interpreting DXA scans, look at the X-rays. These will indicate whether there is any vertebral collapse or a prosthesis present.

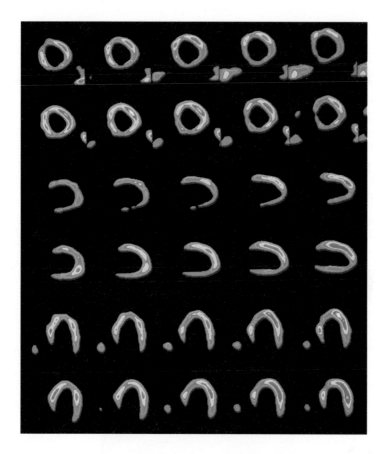

This patient presented with dyspnoea and occasional chest pain.

1. What is this investigation?
2. What does it show?

ANSWERS

1. A ^{99m}Tc–sestamibi cardiac scan. The images are presented in three rows of paired images, the upper row of the pair being the image taken with the patient undergoing pharmacological stress with adenosine, and the lower without stress. The study can be done either on one day or on two separate days. The upper pair is across the short axis of the left ventricle, the middle pair along the vertical long axis and the lower pair along the horizontal long axis.

2. The left ventricle wall is generally thinned and the cavity large. On the stress images there is irregular underperfusion of the inferior wall and septum, and this is largely unchanged in the rest study.

The appearances are those of a dilated cardiomyopathy with extensive small vessel disease. In this case, the underlying cause was an alcoholic cardiomyopathy. A normal study is shown below for comparison.

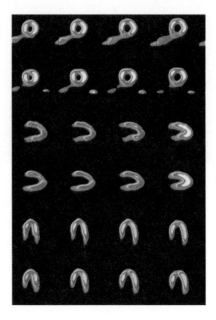

TEACHING POINTS

- One of the main difficulties in interpreting cardiac images is defects caused by attenuation. In females this is seen in the anterior wall and is related to breast attenuation. In males and females who are significantly overweight it can be seen in the inferior wall.
- In asthmatics, dobutamine is used instead of adenosine.

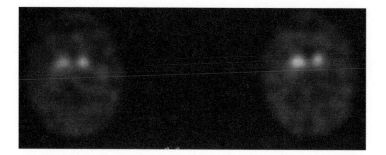

This patient developed tremor and a degree of rigidity. The question posed was whether this was due to Parkinson's disease or essential tremor. The above investigation was performed.

1. What is the investigation?
2. What does it show?

ANSWERS

1. A DAT scan. This is performed using ^{123}I–FP–CIT, a cocaine analogue. It binds to dopamine transfer sites, which are diminished in Parkinson's disease.
2. The scan demonstrates the basal ganglia.

A normal DAT scan is shown below for comparison. The whole of the basal ganglia are shown, with the caudate nucleus anteriorly, leading into the putamen. In Parkinson's disease there is slow loss of activity from the putamen posteriorly and in very severe disease there is no activity in the putamen and hardly any in the caudate nucleus.

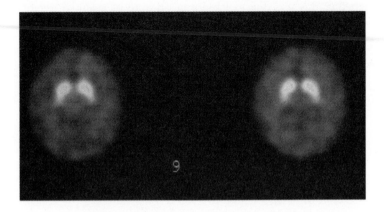

TEACHING POINT

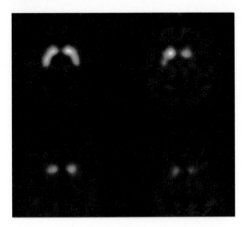

- This scan shows the gradation from normal to severe dopamine transmitter loss in Parkinson's and allows the differentiation between Parkinson's disease, essential tremor and drug-induced tremor. In the latter two conditions the DAT scan is normal.

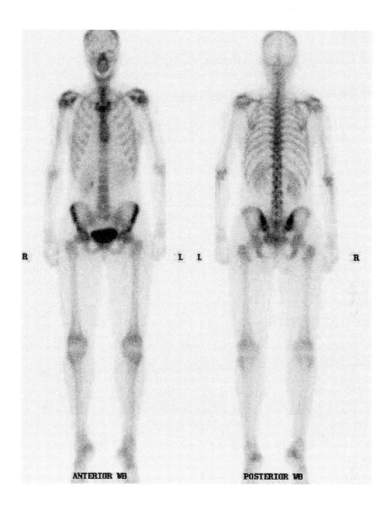

ANTERIOR WB   POSTERIOR WB

1. What does this image show?
2. What tracers may be used?
3. What is the EDE (effective dose equivalent) and DRL (diagnostic reference level)?

ANSWERS

1. This is a normal adult bone scan, showing activity within the skeleton, kidneys and bladder. The major skeletal structures are easily identified. The activity in the sinuses, and the slightly increased activity around the shoulders, are normal.
2. ^{99m}Tc-MDP (methylene diphosphonate) is used in this scan; ^{18}F-fluoride can also be used for bone scanning. Indeed, it was the original tracer used until technetium-labelled diphosphonates became available.
3. A typical injected activity for a planar scan in a 70 kg patient is 600 MBq, with an effective dose of 3 mSv. Should SPECT be considered appropriate, the administered activity may be increased to 800 MBq. The activity may be increased over 600 MBq in extremely large patients or those in pain who need to be scanned quickly. However, if departing from the department's diagnostic reference level (DRL), it is important to ensure the reason for the increased activity is written in the patient's file.

TEACHING POINTS

- The areas nearest the camera faces appear 'hotter' than deeper structures, and fat/muscle attenuates the image and degrades the appearance. The increased uptake seen in the sternomanubrial joint is a normal variant. However, if the patient has breast cancer then there is a significant incidence of a solitary breast metastasis in this region.
- As the isotope is excreted via the kidneys, care must be taken with incontinent patients, and it is obligatory for the referring clinician to inform the department in such cases. It may be advisable to arrange that incontinent patients be catheterized.
- In catheterized patients, the urine within the catheter bag will be radioactive, so appropriate instructions must be given to the nursing staff. With ^{99m}Tc, which has a half-life of 6 h, there is usually not much problem, but should longer half-life isotopes be used, then extra care needs to be taken.

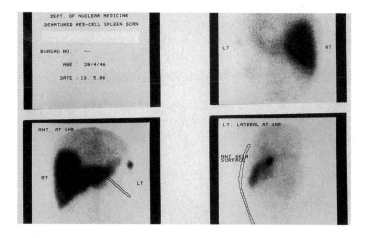

DEPT. OF NUCLEAR MEDICINE
DENATURED RED-CELL SPLEEN SCAN

BUREAU NO. : --

AGE : 20/4/46

DATE : 13. 5.06

LT   RT

ANT. AT 1HR

RT   LT

LT. LATERAL AT 1HR

ANT SKIN
SURFACE

1. What does this study show?
2. What tracer is used?

ANSWERS

1. This is a denatured red cell study used to detect splenunculi. There is a small area of increased uptake at the site of the spleen and this is a recurrent splenunculus. This patient had had a splenectomy for hypersplenism. Several years later, his hypersplenism recurred. The study can also be used to show if there is any functioning splenic tissue after trauma.
2. Red cells are labelled with technetium. The study requires labelled red cells to be heated in order to denature them. They are then naturally trapped in the liver and spleen.

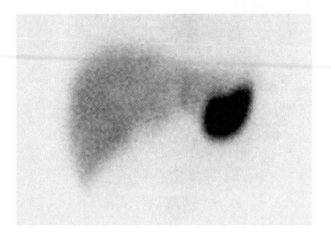

The above case is that of a patient who suffered splenic trauma in a road accident. The question posed was whether there was any functioning splenic tissue, since if not, the patient would need to be on longterm antibiotics.

TEACHING POINT

● Whilst the spleen is usually evaluated using ultrasound or CT, do not forget the value of nuclear medicine imaging when looking for small or ectopic splenic foci.

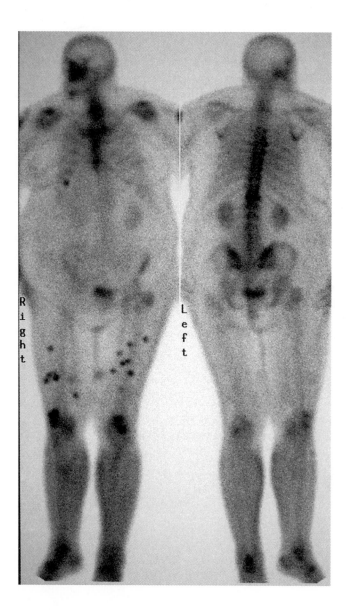

This is the bone scan of a woman.

1. What are the abnormalities?
2. What is the underlying disease she suffers from?

ANSWERS

1. (i) The patient is grossly obese, which makes imaging difficult as the excessive tissues attenuate the photons, giving rise to an unsharp image, and small lesions could easily be missed. (ii) There are a large number of punctate areas of increased uptake in the anterior aspect of both thighs. These are due to injections. (iii) There is increased uptake in L1 and the right 7th rib anteriorly, due to vertebral collapse and a rib fracture. (iv) Osteoarthritis changes are seen in the knees and feet.

2. Type 1 diabetes. The patient regularly injects herself with insulin.

TEACHING POINT

- Any cellular damage due to trauma or infection will give rise to micro-calcifications, and these will be apparent on bone scans. Other non-bone causes of activity include:
  - Urine contamination.
  - Tissued injection.
  - Activity in brain following a cerebrovascular accident.
  - Infarction of brain, heart, lung or spleen (especially in patients with sickle cell disease).
  - Malignant pleural effusions.
  - Osteosarcoma secondaries and other malignancies, e.g. breast and liver deposits.

(A full list may be found in Silberstein E, McAfee J, Spasoff A. *Diagnostic patterns in Nuclear Medicine*. SNM Press, 2000.)

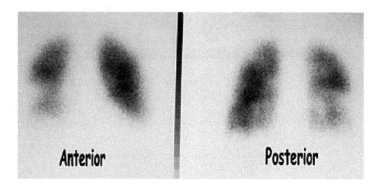

This is a complete study.

1. What is the indication for this study?

ANSWERS

1. This is a lung perfusion scan performed to determine the differential lung function prior to a lobectomy or pneumonectomy.

This study only uses MAA and no ventilation scan is needed. The differential lung function is calculated in a similar manner to that for the differential function for a renal DMSA scan.

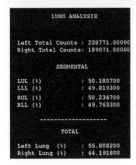

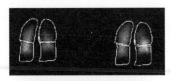

```
              LUNG ANALYSIS


  Left Total Counts : 238771.00000
  Right Total Counts: 189071.00000

                  SEGMENTAL

  LUL (%)            : 50.180700
  LLL (%)            : 49.819300
  RUL (%)            : 50.236700
  RLL (%)            : 49.763300

  ---------------------
                   TOTAL

  Left Lung  (%)     : 55.808200
  Right Lung (%)     : 44.191800
```

TEACHING POINT

- The British Thoracic Society Guidelines on the Fitness for Surgery (www.brit-thoracic.org.uk) advise that if the preoperative FEV1 is <2 L, then a differential lung function study should be performed. If the estimated postoperative FEV1 is <40% of the predicted value, then the surgical risk will be high.

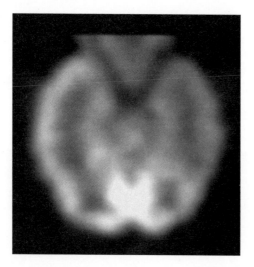

1. What tracer is this?
2. What abnormality does the scan show?
3. What is the clinical indication for this study?

ANSWERS

1. An ¹⁸F-FDG brain scan.
2. It shows reduced uptake in the left temporal lobe compared with the right.
3. Intractable epilepsy in a patient being considered for surgery.

Below is the MRI.

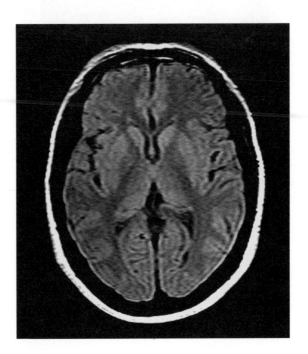

TEACHING POINTS

- The scan is performed interictally to see if there is a region of reduced uptake of FDG, which lateralizes the site of the epileptic focus. PET-FDG scanning is most useful when the clinical, EEG and MRI features do not definitely lateralize the focus.
- The region of reduced uptake is larger than the epileptic focus so the scan is used for lateralization not localization.
- In patients who are having frequent seizures, it may be necessary to perform an EEG during the FDG uptake phase in order to ensure the patient is interictal. If the patient has a seizure during the uptake phase, then the side of the epileptic focus will have increased uptake of FDG.

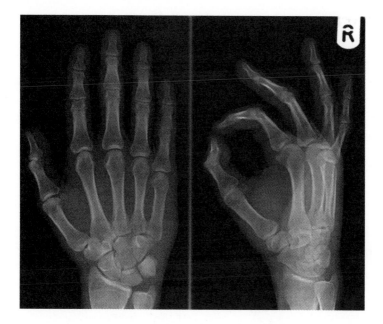

This patient was working on a building site and some scaffolding fell on his hand. This is the casualty X-ray.

1. What can you say about this?
2. What is the next investigation?

ANSWERS

1. No abnormality is seen on the X-ray of the hand (left image) and wrist (right image).
2. A bone scan.

The patient continued to complain of pain in the anatomical snuff box, so he was sent for a bone scan, using ^{99m}Tc-MDP. This shows obvious uptake in the scaphoid, which is typical of a fracture.

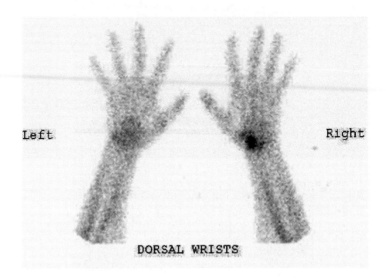

TEACHING POINTS

- The importance of making the diagnosis cannot be stressed too highly, since if a fracture is untreated, the distal pole of the scaphoid may undergo necrosis, as the blood supply is via an end-artery.
- It can take up to 4 days following a fracture for there to be sufficient bone reaction to make the scan positive. It is important not to scan the patient too soon and thus get a false negative.
- Whenever there is a clinical query about a scaphoid fracture, a bone scan is the investigation of choice, as it is quicker, easier and less costly than an MRI of the wrist (which would also demonstrate the fracture).

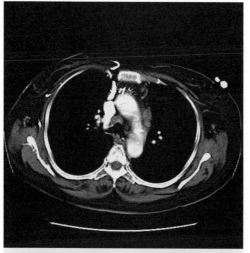

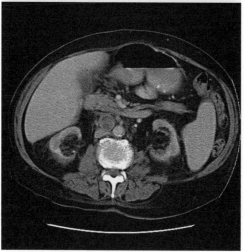

This patient had previously been treated for tuberculosis, but remained unwell with raised inflammatory markers. The CT images were unchanged over several months.

1. What can be seen?
2. What investigations would you do next?

ANSWERS

1. Abnormal tissue in the hilar and mediastinal areas, and a large right-sided para-aortic nodal mass with inhomogeneous central low attenuation. This could represent a tuberculous node.
2. A ^{99m}Tc–HMPAO-labelled white cell scan to identify if the abnormalities seen on the CT are infective.

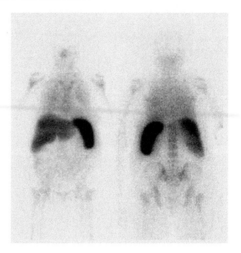

The above images show no areas of increased uptake at the sites seen on CT. The possibility was then raised that the enlarged hilar and para-aortic nodes were due to lymphoma and a PET scan was performed, which showed markedly increased uptake at the left hilum and in the para-aortic region on both sides, indicating active disease.

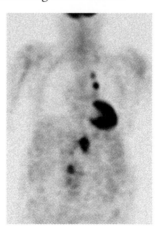

TEACHING POINT

- PET cannot differentiate between inflammation and tumour (in this case tuberculosis or lymphoma), so biopsy with histology and microbiology is needed to make the final diagnosis. In this case, biopsy of the para-aortic nodes is easiest.

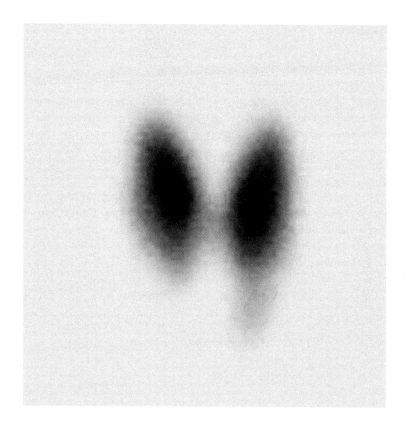

This patient suffered from tiredness, weight loss and insomnia.

1. What is your diagnosis?
2. What else could you do?

ANSWERS

1. The image shows extremely active uptake within the thyroid, but no background activity. This is typical of Graves' disease. The clue on the pertechnetate scan is that there is very low background, indicating marked uptake of tracer by the thyroid. (Some centres also give a percentage uptake value, based on the administered dose, but this is of little value and bears no relationship to the dose of ^{131}I given for treatment.)

2. The diagnosis of thyrotoxicosis is made clinically and biochemically, with a suppressed TSH, and high FT_4 and FT_3. The role of the isotope scan is to define the type of thyrotoxicosis. Other causes are toxic nodules and Hashimoto's thyroiditis (subacute viral thyroiditis). It is important to differentiate these as treatment will be different from that for Graves'. Toxic nodules may be autonomous, as below, suppressing the rest of the gland.

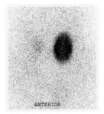

In cases of toxic nodules, there is obvious uptake, and with time these nodules may suppress the rest of the gland and become autonomous. In Hashimoto's, there is no uptake despite the biochemical thyrotoxicosis, and the disease is self-limiting, gradually returning to normal.

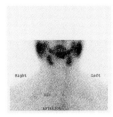

TEACHING POINT

- Where there is biochemical evidence of thyrotoxicosis, a pertechnetate scan is extremely useful in differentiating the cause and guiding treatment.

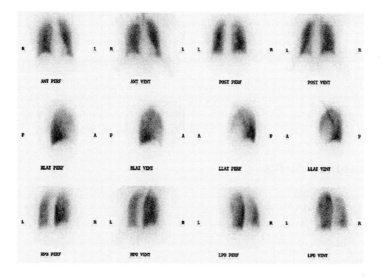

ANT PERF   ANT VENT   POST PERF   POST VENT

RLAT PERF   RLAT VENT   LLAT PERF   LLAT VENT

RPO PERF   RPO VENT   LPO PERF   LPO VENT

1. What does this image show?

ANSWER

1. This is a normal lung scan, showing both perfusion and ventilation scans, as matched pairs.

The scans are obtained in anterior, posterior, LPO, RPO and lateral views. The perfusion and ventilation scans may be obtained at the same time, using dual isotope acquisition programs, or one after the other. The ventilation images can be identified by the ^{81m}Kr in the trachea on the anterior view.

TEACHING POINTS

- The perfusion scan uses ^{99m}Tc-labelled microspheres, which must be agitated in the syringe prior to injection to prevent clumping and injected with the patient supine.
- ^{81m}Kr has a half-life of 13 s, making it the ideal ventilation agent.
- Other agents can be used to provide ventilation images. ^{133}Xe gas (half-life 5.25 h) is widely used in the US and was used in the PIOPED study, but not the UK because of contamination issues, high dose to the operators and poor image quality. Also, three sets of images are obtained – inspiration, equilibrium and washout. This means that the length of time for the study is great. Normally only posterior views are obtained, although with double-headed cameras, anterior views are possible.
- A ^{99m}Tc-labelled aerosol of DTPA, which can be inhaled, is often used in the UK. However, this isotope is used to demonstrate the perfusion (^{99m}Tc-labelled MAA microspheres), and it is not advisable to use the same isotope for the perfusion and ventilation images at the same time. Caution should be exercised with ^{99m}Tc-DTPA aerosol to avoid room and camera contamination, if sucked into the gamma-camera head by fans. ^{99m}Tc has a half-life of 6 h, so a contaminated camera is effectively out of action for 24 h.
- Pulmonary hypertension is a relative contraindication to V/Q scanning, as the particles block a small percentage (<1%) of the small arterioles. In patients with pulmonary hypertension, there is a possibility that the sudden occlusion of even a small number of arterioles could tip the patient into acute right heart failure and death. If no more than 200 000 particles are injected, the examination is safe, and so it is important to know how many particles are given when the perfusion study is performed. Remember that towards the expiry time of the vial of MAA there will be more particles injected per MBq. (This has been well documented by Barrington S, O'Doherty M. Nuc Med Comm 1995; **16**: 125–7.)

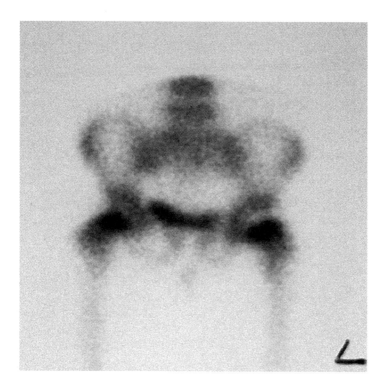

1. What does this bone scan show?
2. What is the significance of this?

ANSWERS

1. A photon-deficient area in the head of the left femur.
2. This is due to diminished vascularity of the femoral head, which can lead to avascular necrosis or Perthe's disease.

The image is a simple anterior view, but if there is any doubt, the hips should be imaged with a pinhole collimator as this gives improved resolution. Positioning is also important. The X-ray may be normal in the early stages of Perthe's disease and only show the typical flattening of the femoral capital epiphysis late, as seen below.

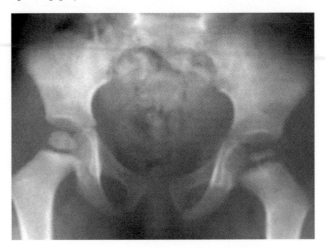

A pinhole image of the hip is shown below. The photopenic area in the proximal femoral epiphysis is typical of Perthe's disease.

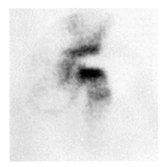

TEACHING POINTS

- The significance of nuclear medicine scanning is that the alterations in blood flow will occur long before there are any X-ray changes. As the initial problem is with venous return from the femoral head, once the abnormal blood flow and thus diminished activity is seen on the bone scan, rapid treatment can be instituted before there is any damage to the femoral head.
- A wide selection of paediatric nuclear medicine cases may be found at www.medical-atlas.org.

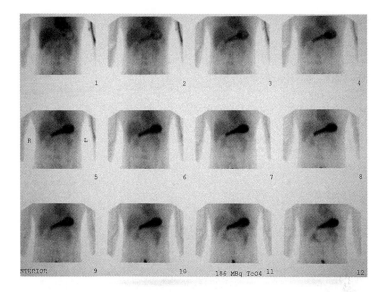

This 24-year-old patient suffered from repeated attacks of anaemia. Endoscopy, both upper and lower, was unhelpful, as were barium studies. The patient was referred for isotope imaging.

1. What is the study and how is it performed?
2. What does the scan show and what is your diagnosis?

ANSWERS

1. This is a scan looking for a Meckel's diverticulum. It is carried out by injecting pertechnetate and imaging sequentially in 5-min frames.
2. The pertechnetate accumulates in functioning gastric mucosa, and so with time the stomach is seen. In addition, a focus of increased activity is seen at the very bottom of the image set, which is activity in a Meckel's diverticulum.

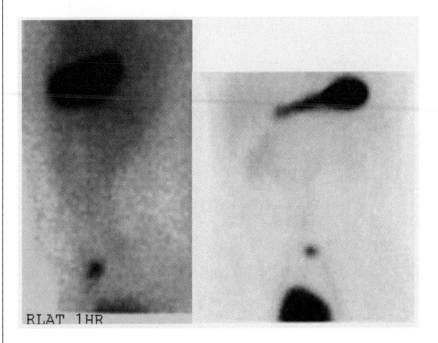

The above views confirm the presence of the Meckel's diverticulum, which is quite separate from the bladder and urinary tract. The Meckel's diverticulum was removed at surgery.

TEACHING POINTS

- It is necessary to pretreat the patient with cimetidine to reduce gastric uptake.
- Meckel's diverticula containing functioning gastric mucosa are those that bleed; Meckel's with no gastric mucosa do not bleed. Demonstration of a Meckel's on a barium follow through study will not indicate those containing gastric mucosa.
- Images should be centred to include the stomach and bladder, and a lateral view obtained at 1 h to demonstrate diverticula lying behind the bladder and invisible on anterior images. Time–activity curves can be drawn to aid the differentiation of renal or bladder activity from gastric mucosa.

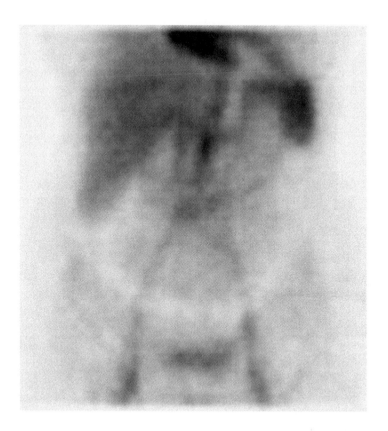

1. What is this scan?
2. What is it for?
3. What else can be seen?

ANSWERS

1. This is a labelled red cell scan, using an injection of stannous chloride followed 20 min later by ^{99m}Tc as pertechnetate, which labels the red cells in vivo.
2. The scan is performed to demonstrate sites of blood loss, especially in the GI tract. Images are performed dynamically for an hour, and areas of blood loss show as sites of increased activity. Delayed images may need to be obtained.
3. This image shows normal distribution within the blood vessels, heart, liver and spleen, but there is a crescentic area of low attenuation across the lower abdomen. This is barium in the colon, from a barium examination the previous day.

TEACHING POINTS

- Metal artefacts can obscure parts of the image. Barium in the bowel is not commonly seen; more usual are prostheses and pacemakers.
- Pharmacological interactions must also be considered. Uptake of radio-iodine in the thyroid, either for diagnosis or therapy, will be adversely affected if the patient has had a radiological intravenous contrast study. Similarly, if the patient has had coffee prior to a pharmacological cardiac stress study, the caffeine will inhibit the vasodilatation caused by the adenosine or dobutamine.
- Thought must be given to the order in which all investigations are requested and performed.
- Other iatrogenic artefacts seen on bone scans are:
  - Increased renal cortical uptake following chemotherapy.
  - Reduced tracer uptake following radiotherapy.
  - Post-surgery the bone scan may show increased uptake for up to a year. This is a clinical problem in infected sternotomy wounds, and the referrer may not think to give any surgical history on the request form, so vital clinical information will be missing. Similarly, the referrer may omit a history of fractures, which may also show increased uptake for up to a year.

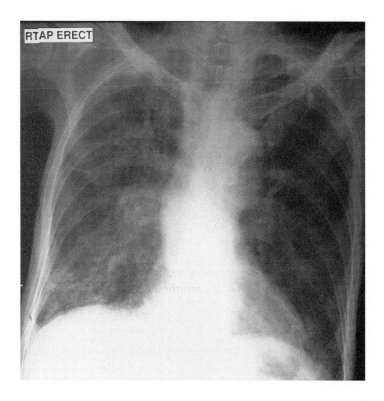

This patient presented with a cough and generalized pains. This is the chest X-ray.

1. What does it show?
2. How else would you investigate the patient?

ANSWERS

1. A soft enlargement of the lower pole of the right hilum and some distal consolidation. This patient is also very thin. The most likely diagnosis is carcinoma of the lung, and this was confirmed on bronchoscopy.
2. Further investigations to stage the disease are bone scanning and liver ultrasound, as shown below.

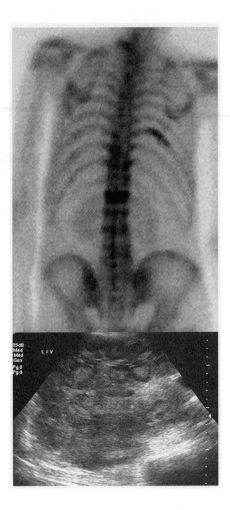

These show the multiple bone and liver deposits. Thus, the patient has stage IV disease and the therapeutic options are chemotherapy with palliative radiotherapy as required. CT scanning of the chest, abdomen and pelvis was also carried out.

TEACHING POINTS

- Lung cancer is common and increasing, and constitutes 22% of all cancers in men and 8% in women. Non-small cell tumours may be curable, so early and accurate diagnosis is crucial.
- Diagnosis is made by biopsy, with staging using CT and ultrasound. Bone scanning is not indicated in the routine staging of patients with lung cancer, but if the patient has bone pain or a raised alkaline phosphatase, it may be indicated.
- [18]FDG-PET scans are used in the staging of patients with potentially operable non-small cell lung cancer since it allows detection of the primary tumour, lymph node stations and distant metastases all in one test. The PET scan below, from another case, shows the intense uptake in a left apical lesion with uptake in right hilar nodes. This information immediately makes the lesion non-operable.

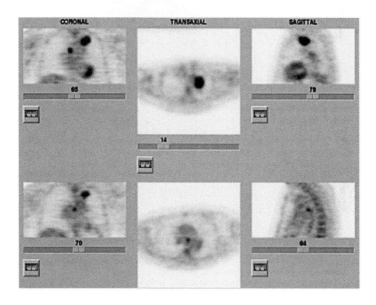

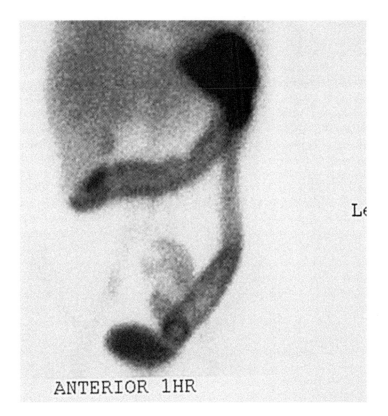

Le

ANTERIOR 1HR

A patient with bloody diarrhoea and a diagnosis of Crohn's disease on colonoscopy needs investigation, and the above image was obtained.

1. What is it and how is it performed?
2. What is its value?

ANSWERS

1. A labelled white cell scan, using ^{99m}Tc-labelled HMPAO. Blood is taken from the patient, spun down and the white cells are labelled with ^{99m}Tc-HMPAO. These are washed and re-injected (this whole process takes about 3 h) and images may be obtained at 1, 2 and 3 h post-injection.
2. ^{99m}Tc-labelled HMPAO is used to demonstrate areas of inflammatory change, and so shows the extent of the disease. In this case there is obvious extensive active Crohn's disease. (There is also a transplanted kidney in the left iliac fossa.)

This test is superior to the conventional barium enema (below), which may continue to look abnormal even if the disease is not active.

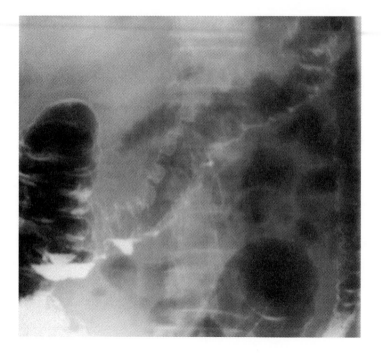

TEACHING POINTS

- The effective dose equivalent from a ^{99m}Tc–HMPAO image (3 mSv) is considerably less than that from a barium enema (7–10 mSv). Colonoscopy has no radiation risk, but in active disease there is a risk of perforating the bowel, possibly with fatal consequences.
- ^{99m}Tc–HMPAO is excreted into the bowel, but not until about 3 h post-injection, so images can be obtained up to 3 h without physiological excretion compromising the images. Thus, if the object of the test is to define inflammatory bowel disease, ^{99m}Tc–HMPAO-labelled white cells can be used, but if the question is that of infection, ^{111}In-labelled white cells need to be used, but for the latter the effective dose to the patient is higher at 9 mSv.

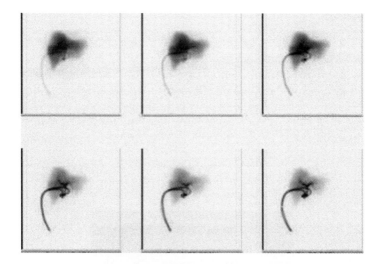

This patient had recently had a complicated abdominal operation, necessitating the placing of a drain. This set of images was obtained from a dynamic series.

1. What is the examination?
2. What does it show and why?

ANSWERS

1. A HIDA scan. HIDA, labelled with ^{99m}Tc, is excreted by the liver in the same way as bilirubin, and so can be used to show the biliary tree.
2. This case shows normal liver uptake and visualization of the biliary tree, but total block of the common bile duct and filling of a drain to the right. There is also accumulation of activity in the gallbladder bed. This indicates a total block of the common bile duct, and leakage from the stump of the cystic duct.

The patient had had a laparascopic cholecystectomy, converted to an open operation. The CT below shows that numerous clips have been placed in the gallbladder bed, including one across the common bile duct.

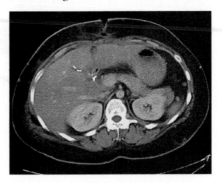

A normal HIDA scan is shown below. This clearly shows the progression of activity through the liver, into the biliary tree and gallbladder, and then into the small bowel.

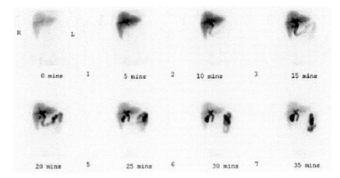

TEACHING POINTS

- Because the cystic duct is patent, the gallbladder is shown on the normal HIDA scan.
- In the past the HIDA test was used in cases of suspected acute cholecystitis, as in this condition oedema closes off the cystic duct and therefore the gallbladder is not visualized. The HIDA scan was >95% sensitive and specific in acute cholecystitis. However, HIDA has been superseded by ultrasound in the diagnosis of acute cholecystitis and is now only used to visualize the biliary tree post-surgery and to investigate post-surgical leaks.

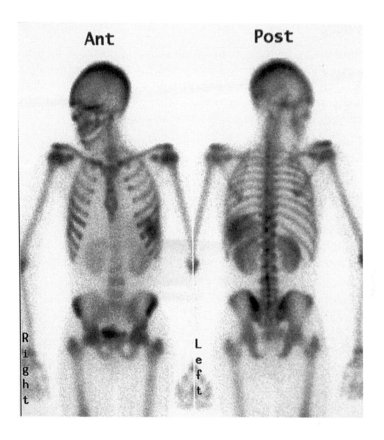

This patient presented with generalized aches and pains, with more marked pain in the left upper quadrant. This is the bone scan.

1. What does it show?
2. What is the disease?

ANSWERS

1. Normal bones, but there is an area of increased uptake in the left upper quadrant above the kidney. This is activity in the spleen.
2. Sickle cell anaemia, which may present with bone pain and infarcts, although not in this case. There are often splenic micro-infarcts, which calcify, allowing them to be visualized on a bone scan.

TEACHING POINTS

- As well as areas of increased uptake within the long bones due to infarcts, there may also be evidence of avascular necrosis of the joints in sickle cell anaemia. Soft tissue uptake may be seen in the lungs, due to infarction, and the kidneys may be more prominent.
- The clinical problem is often the differentiation of a bone infarct from infection. In both of these situations, the bone scan will be 'hot'.

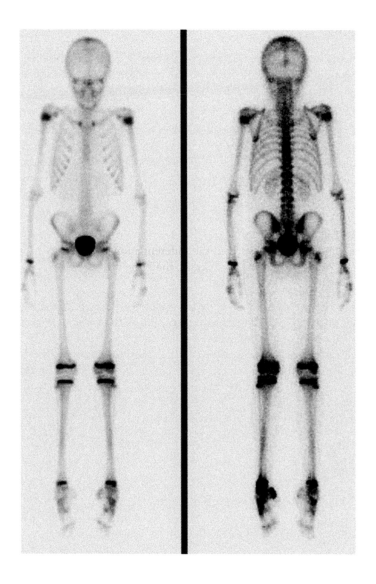

1. What does this image show?

ANSWER

1. This is a normal paediatric bone scan using ^{99m}Tc–MDP, showing activity within the skeleton, kidneys and bladder. The epiphyseal growth plates show increased activity, as they are sites of increased bone turnover.

A typical injected activity for a planar scan in a 70 kg patient is 600 MBq, with appropriate reductions for children. The reduction in dose may be determined either by age or by weight (the Administration of Radioactive Substances Advisory Committee [ARSAC] has published tables to allow you to determine the dose).

TEACHING POINTS

- In children, the skull vault appears larger than the facial bones. Facial bones are generally metabolically more active than the vault as they grow at a faster rate.
- It is important that the whole of the skeleton is imaged. This image was taken on a whole-body gamma camera, although a series of static images may be obtained, depending on the situation.
- In all cases, it is helpful to try to get the child to empty his/her bladder immediately prior to imaging. However, in small children this may not be possible and it may be necessary to mask the activity within the bladder electronically.
- Sedation is rarely required in paediatric cases.

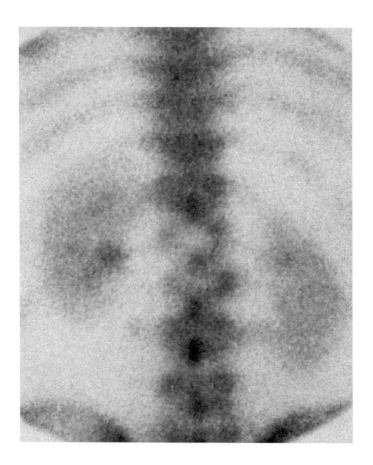

This patient presented with back pain and, as there was the suspicion of malignancy, a bone scan was requested.

1. What does it show?
2. What is the disease?

ANSWERS

1. A large photopenic area on the right side of L2.
2. There is either no blood reaching that part of the vertebra or an osteoclastic process is occurring. Osteoclastic processes do not excite bone reaction and so are not seen on conventional bone scans. Large osteoclastic lesions are seen as 'cold' areas, as here. The patient has a solitary plasmacytoma.

The X-ray (below) only showed minimal porosis of the vertebra.

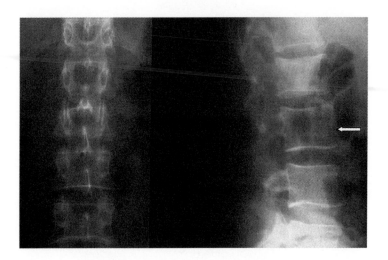

TEACHING POINTS

- Plasmacytoma and myeloma are not shown on bone scans, unless the deposits are very large or they fracture. Once they fracture, normal osteoblastic processes occur, and so the healing fracture is seen on a bone scan.
- The diagnosis is made by satisfying two of the following three criteria:
    - Presence of neoplastic plasma cells in bone marrow aspirate.
    - Abnormal M band γ-globulin on electrophoresis.
    - Radiological evidence of bone destruction or profound osteoporosis.

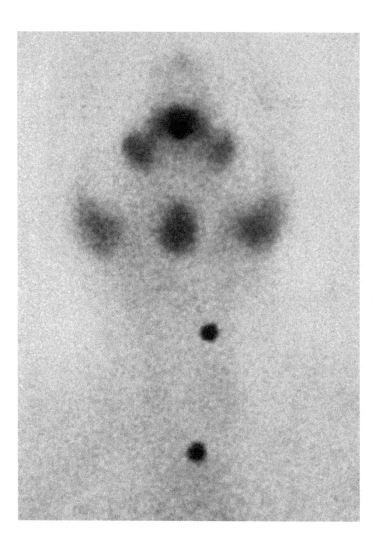

This child had the above investigation.

1. What is it?
2. What does it show?

ANSWERS

1. A thyroid scan using ^{99m}Tc as pertechnetate.
2. The markers represent the thyroid cartilage and the sternal notch. There is uptake in the salivary glands, which are normal, but there is no thyroid activity. However, there is a focus of intense activity in the midline. This is not normally seen and represents a lingual thyroid.

Confirmation is obtained from a lateral view (below). This shows uptake in the buccal mucosa and salivary glands, and the back of the tongue, confirming a lingual thyroid. The markers represent tip of chin and thyroid cartilage. Clinically, this patient presented with a smooth red swelling at the back of the tongue.

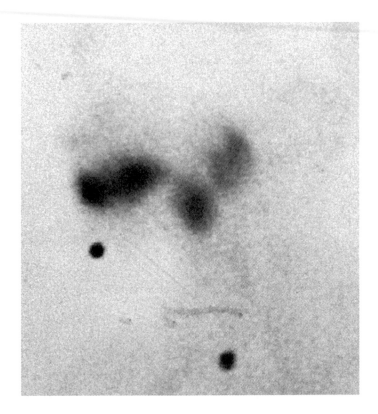

TEACHING POINT

- Whenever a patient presents with a smooth swelling at the base of the tongue, a thyroid scan should be performed to identify a lingual thyroid. This is especially important in children; should the swelling be removed without imaging, the child will lose all thyroid tissue and become hypothyroid.

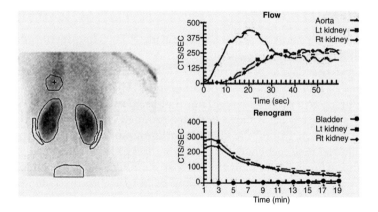

1. What is this investigation and how is it performed?
2. What does it show?
3. What additional drugs may be given and when?

ANSWERS

1. A MAG3 dynamic renogram labelled with ^{99m}Tc. The patient presented with renal pain, and the ultrasound showed rather full collecting systems, suggesting a degree of obstruction. To stress the kidneys, furosemide is given 10 min prior to the MAG3 injection. The furosemide dose is 0.5 mg/kg up to a maximum of 40 mg. This is known as an F–10 renogram.

2. This scan is normal. It shows (left), the summed view with the regions of interest drawn around the kidneys, background, heart and bladder. The computer then generates two sets of background subtracted curves (right). The upper set shows the clearance through the heart and into the kidneys. There is symmetrical inflow of isotope into the kidneys. The lower graph shows the uptake and clearance of isotope and no evidence of obstruction. The two parallel lines between 2 and 3 min are the conventional time when the relative function is calculated. Function should be 50%/50% ± 5%. Furosemide is used to ensure there is an adequate diuresis when the tracer is given.

3. In cases of suspected renal artery stenosis as a cause of hypertension, two renograms are performed, one without and one with a low dose of captopril (an ACE inhibitor) being given. In functional renal artery stenosis there is vasoconstriction of the efferent arteriole in the renal glomerulus. This helps maintain glomerular filtration. Captopril dilates this arteriole and thus reduces the filtration pressure in the glomerulus and thus the filtration rate. This results in a worsening of the renogram curve on the affected side. Unilateral disease may be simple to demonstrate, but bilateral disease may be more complicated.

TEACHING POINTS

- Dynamic renograms may be performed with ^{99m}Tc-labelled DTPA or MAG3. MAG3 is better, giving a higher target/background ratio.
- In any case of suspected obstruction, a stress renogram with furosemide challenge should be performed.
- In children, furosemide may be given just before the injection of MAG3 to avoid either two punctures, or leaving a cannula in needlessly. This is known as an F0 renogram.
- For children the activity of ^{99m}Tc administered is reduced, and calculated either by age or weight. (Administration of Radioactive Substances Advisory Committee [ARSAC] has published tables to allow you to do this.) The dose of furosemide is also reduced, based on the weight of the child.

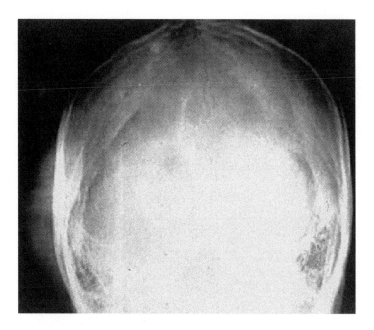

This child presented with a fairly hard painful lump on the lateral aspect of the head, and no history of trauma. The lump had appeared rather quickly.

1. What can you see?

ANSWER

1. An area of rather dense soft tissue swelling over the left parietal bone, with no obvious underlying bony abnormality. The sutures are fused, so this is not a caput following birth trauma. There is some spiculation within the lesion, but no obvious underlying bone destruction.

The speed of progress and pain are suggestive of a malignant lesion, and in a child this could either be a primary bone neoplasm such as an osteo-sarcoma, which has a peak incidence between ages 10 and 20 years, or a secondary from a primary such as a Wilms' tumour. A bone scan was performed.

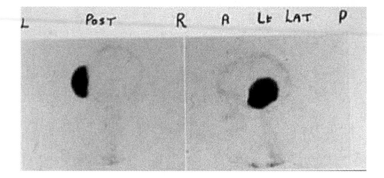

This shows an intensely metabolically active lesion, suppressing activity in the rest of the skull. The rest of the skeleton was normal, making secondaries unlikely.

TEACHING POINTS

- The bone scan shows an area of intense bone metabolic activity, and is therefore due to malignancy, but the scan is non-specific.
- Osteosarcomas commonly arise in the metaphyseal region of the distal femur or proximal tibia, but are also seen in the proximal humerus and pelvis. They often present with a fracture. Lesions in the skull or other bones are rarer. The tumours metastasize early and pulmonary metastases are a cause of uptake in the lungs on a bone scan.
- Multifocal osteosarcomas may occur and these will show abnormal uptake at several sites in the skeleton, but are difficult to differentiate from metastases.

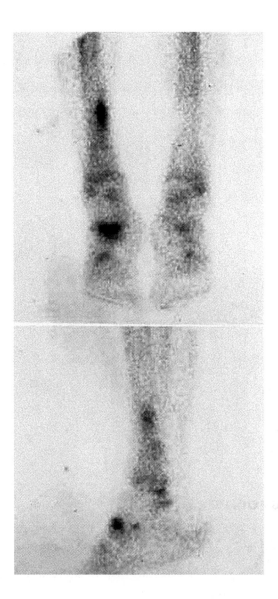

This teenager liked sport and was good at long jumping. After an event, he complained of leg pain. He had not sustained any trauma directly to the leg recently. Above is the bone scan of his lower limbs.

1. What can you see?

ANSWER

1. An area of increased uptake in the mid–right tibia and in the tarsus on the right, probably at the talo–navicular joint. The tibial uptake is abnormal and with this history represents a stress fracture. The tarsal uptake may also represent a stress fracture, but early degenerative change in an athlete is more likely.

This X-ray of the lower tibia is normal, but confirms the early talo–navicular osteoarthritis.

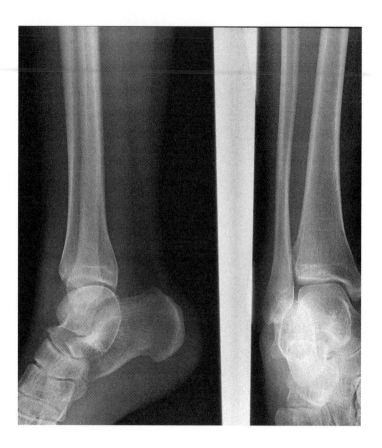

TEACHING POINT

- X-rays are very insensitive in detecting cortical microfractures, and where there is a good history, a bone scan is much more sensitive and should be requested early. A positive bone scan allows rapid, appropriate treatment.

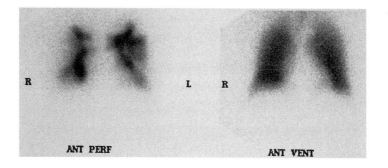

R   L   R

ANT PERF   ANT VENT

This patient presented with shortness of breath and a normal chest X-ray. The next investigation was a lung scan.

1. What does this show?
2. What would you do next?
3. How would you manage the case?

ANSWERS

1. Typical segmental perfusion defects with a normal ventilation pattern, typical of pulmonary emboli.
2. A contrast helical CT.
3. Anticoagulate the patient, initially with low molecular weight heparin, proceeding to full warfarinisation.

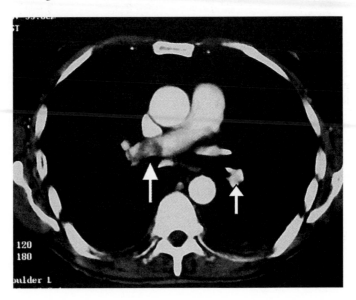

This showed the clot sitting in the right main pulmonary artery and left lower lobe artery. Whilst an extremely useful investigation, CT will only show clot in the first few branches of the pulmonary arteries.

TEACHING POINTS

- The main problem with V/Q scans is the high number of intermediate probability scans. This problem can be partially answered by performing CT pulmonary angiography (CPTA) in those patients who have an abnormal chest X-ray. (There is some debate about whether all patients with a suspected pulmonary embolism should have CTPA.) However, CPTA will show other lung pathologies.
- It should be remembered that a normal V/Q scan excludes pulmonary embolism. Thus, in those patients in whom the pre-test likelihood of pulmonary embolism is low and who have a normal chest X-ray, a V/Q scan will give an answer in most patients with a lower radiation burden.
- Remember that other lung pathologies can occur with the same risk factors. Do not forget pneumothorax as a cause of pleuritic chest pain in young people.
- It is good practice to perform a repeat lung scan once the patient has been treated and anticoagulated, to obtain a baseline post-treatment scan should the patient re-present.

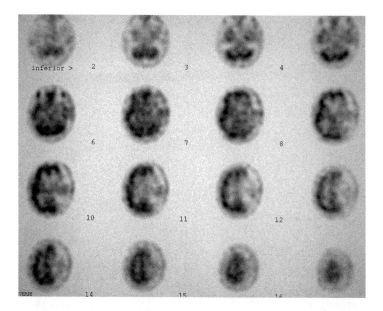

This patient had several small intracranial aneurysms shown on cerebral angiography, and they were clipped. After surgery, there was some weakness noted on the right and the above examination was performed.

1. What is the examination?
2. What does it show?

ANSWERS

1. An HMPAO brain scan.
2. Cerebral blood flow. There is a large left-sided defect, indicating markedly diminished flow in the middle cerebral artery territory.

A normal brain HMPAO scan is shown below.

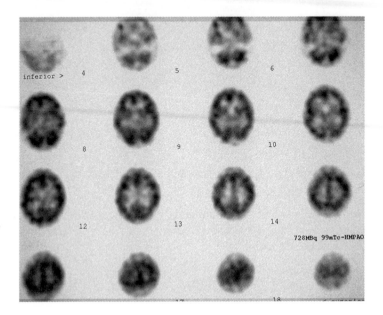

inferior >   4   5   6

8   9   10

12   13   14

728MBq 99mTc-HMPAO

TEACHING POINTS

- HMPAO brain scans are extremely sensitive in showing alteration of cerebral blood flow, and are positive long before any changes are seen on CT or even MRI in patients with acute cerebral events. However, at present there is little active acute management of these conditions and thus the clinical relevance is uncertain.
- HMPAO brain scans are sometimes used in other cerebral diseases, e.g. dementias.

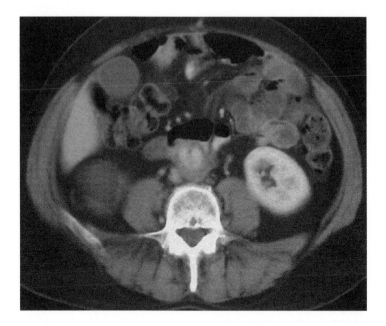

This patient recently underwent an aortic graft, and post-operatively was ill with fever, pain and a high C-reactive protein. Above is the contrast CT.

1. What other imaging modalities might help?

ANSWER

1. The CT clearly shows a collection around the aorta, but it is impossible to say if it is infected. The next study was a ^{99m}Tc-labelled HMPAO white cell image (below), looking for a source of infection.

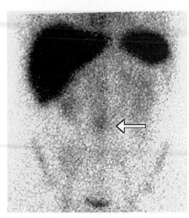

This shows an area of increased uptake in the mid-abdomen (arrow), just below the kidneys, which suggests infection round the graft. To confirm this, a PET scan using the glucose analogue ^{18}FDG was carried out (below). ^{18}FDG is taken up in areas of infection, as well as in tumours. There is also normal ^{18}FDG accumulation in the bladder and right colon.

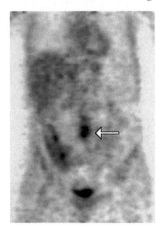

TEACHING POINTS

- CT shows the anatomy, but isotope imaging shows the foci of infection required by the surgeon, as a re-operation after graft surgery is extremely difficult and hazardous.
- Radionuclide studies differ from X-ray, MRI and ultrasound in that it is the function that is being imaged. This is often of clinical importance in assessing the radiological abnormalities. Labelled white cells and FDG indicate local inflammation and it is only in conjunction with the clinical and radiological picture that diagnosis of an infected graft can be made.

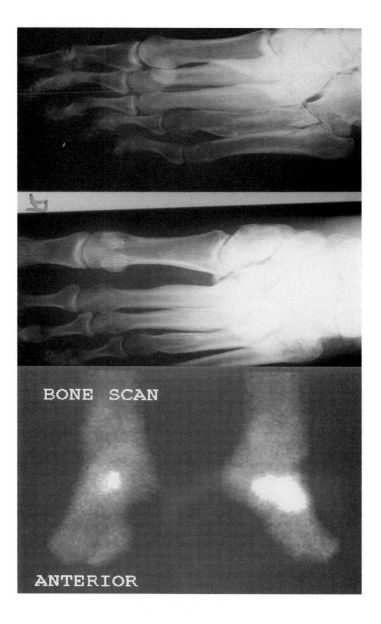

This 24-year-old female diabetic presented with a hot swollen foot and fevers. The putative diagnosis was osteomyelitis.

1. What do these images show?
2. Do they diagnose osteomyelitis?
3. How would you continue the investigations?

ANSWERS

1. A disorganized tarsus with old periosteal reactions along the metatarsals, typical of a Charcot joint in a diabetic. The bone scan image is a late static image of the feet. Often the uptake in the feet is relatively poor and low quality images are obtained. This is why the image looks like a blood pool image. In suspected infection, it is useful to take a blood pool image since the presence of increased blood pool activity with a normal bone scan confirms soft tissue infection or inflammation. The first pass blood flow image is mentioned in some books but most units do not acquire this image since it adds little to the case.

2. No. In the diagnosis of osteomyelitis, bone scans are very sensitive. In the presence of a normal X-ray they are also very specific. However, the difficulty arises when the bones are abnormal, as in this case. Under these circumstances the bone scan specificity is low and this means that it is unlikely to be of help. Other infection imaging agents can help, but they may not have sufficient resolution to enable the differentiation of soft tissue infection from osteomyelitis.

3. Further investigations useful in diagnosing osteomyelitis are:
   - Leukoscan – a ^{99m}Tc-labelled monoclonal antibody to white cells, raised in mice. It labels areas of increased white cell concentration.

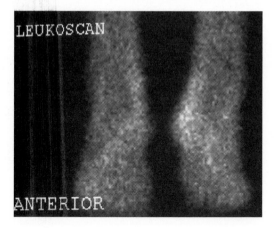

- ^{99m}Tc-labelled HMPAO (Exametazime) white cells. These show areas of increased white cell concentration.

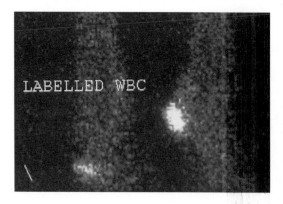

These two images show that there is no uptake in the tarsus, which excludes the diagnosis of osteomyelitis. There is, however, uptake in the heel, best seen on the HMPAO scan, and this was due to a superficial ulcer.

TEACHING POINTS

- X-rays are often unhelpful and a bone scan is only valuable when negative.
- Leukoscan does not involve handling blood products, unlike HMPAO, so there is no risk to the radiopharmacist of hepatitis B or C, or HIV. The labelling is also easier and does not require closed cabinets, so it can be used in smaller departments, or in departments remote from a full radio-pharmacy.
- White cells can be labelled with ^{99m}Tc or ^{111}In.
- As diabetics are at increased risk of osteomyelitis, especially in Charcot joints, ruling out osteomyelitis avoids amputation.

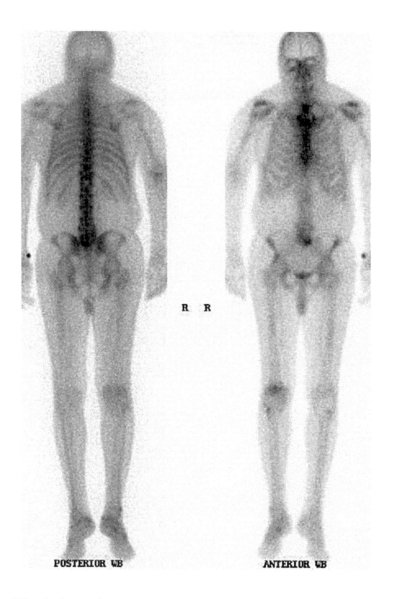

R R

POSTERIOR WB   ANTERIOR WB

1. What is the scan?
2. What does it show?

ANSWERS

1. A whole body bone scan.
2. Some slight increased uptake at L5, typical of degenerative disease. However, the kidneys and bladder are not seen, and the background is higher than normal for a thin patient.

This patient has chronic renal failure, so there is no renal excretion of bone agent.

TEACHING POINTS

- Remember that more than the skeleton is demonstrated on a bone scan, and renal tract or soft tissue lesions can also be diagnosed, as in this case.
- The differential might be a 'superscan' in extensive skeletal metastatic disease. In renal failure the background is high, which rules out extensive skeletal metastases or metabolic bone disease. In a superscan (below) the bony uptake is increased to such an extent that relatively little tracer is excreted renally. This explains why the background is low, the renal tract is not well seen and the bone uptake is increased. Remember that in normal situations, approximately 30% of the diphosphonate is excreted renally.

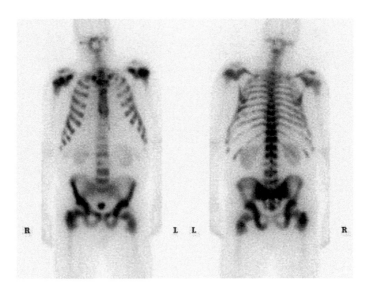

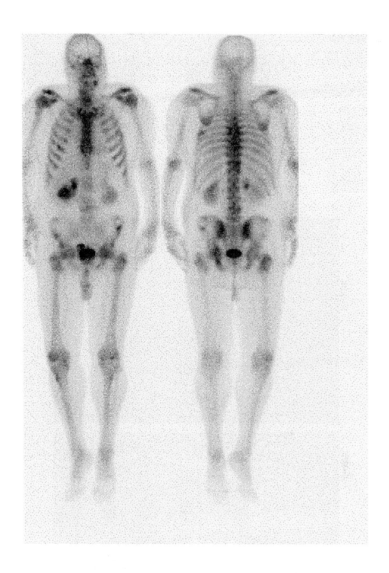

1. What abnormalities does this bone scan show?
2. Suggest a unifying diagnosis.

ANSWERS

1. A low grade increased uptake in the right 6th rib anteriorly and in the left 8th rib posteriorly. There is also some increased uptake in T6 or 7. There is an unusual shape to the right kidney.
2. The renal abnormality suggests a renal carcinoma with bone metastases. An alternative would be a carcinoma with both bone and renal metastases.

Ultrasound and CT will aid in the diagnosis. These images clearly show the lesion in the right kidney, and the appearances are those of a renal cell carcinoma.

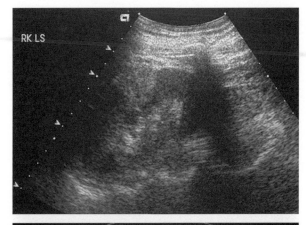

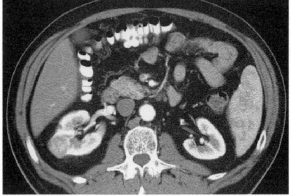

TEACHING POINT

- Remember in bone scans to look at the renal tract and other regions of soft tissue uptake. The scan below shows renal uptake in a patient with sickle cell disease (or in other contexts hypercalcaemia or post-chemotherapy). Uptake is seen in the left lung base as well. A focus is also seen in the right midfemur on the anterior but not the posterior view, indicating that it is an artefact.

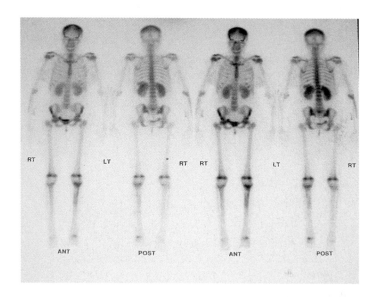

RT LT RT RT LT RT

ANT POST ANT POST

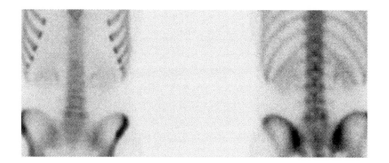

This young sportsman presented to the team doctor with low back pain. The plain X-rays are normal.

1. What does this image show?
2. What other imaging would be useful?

ANSWERS

1. A ⁹⁹ᵐTc-MDP planar bone scan, which shows minimally increased uptake in the pedicles of L5, but no diagnosis could be made from this study.
2. A tomographic study. This is known as SPECT (single photon emission CT), which is the nuclear medicine version of conventional CT. The data is acquired with the camera heads rotating around the patient, and then reconstituted in sagittal, coronal and transverse planes.

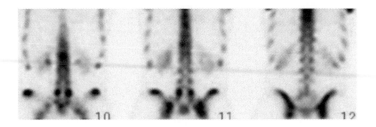

These coronal images clearly show that there is abnormal uptake in the pedicles, and the likeliest diagnosis is that of bilateral pars fractures. These were confirmed on CT (arrows).

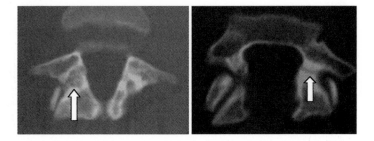

TEACHING POINTS

● The anatomy of pars fractures is best shown on CT or MRI, but these cannot indicate whether the lesion is recent. Improved localisation aids specificity of interpretation. Facet joint lesions are benign.
● Increased uptake on the bone scan confirms either a recent fracture or continued instability.
● This combination of anatomical imaging (CT or MRI) with physiological imaging (bone scan) is the most useful for the clinician.

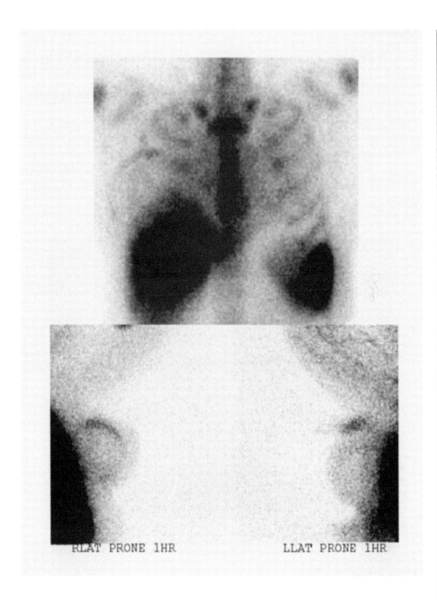

RLAT PRONE 1HR   LLAT PRONE 1HR

This patient had pain in the right side of the chest anteriorly, fever and a raised white cell count after an operation.

1. What tracer is used and what other tracers might be considered?
2. What does the image show and what operation had the patient undergone?
3. What imaging would you do next?

ANSWERS

1. A labelled white cell scan, using ^{99m}Tc-labelled HMPAO, looking for sites of infection. ^{111}In can also be used for labelling HMPAO, and because there is no bowel or urinary activity, this agent is ideal in cases of suspected intra-abdominal sepsis. Leukoscan, a ^{99m}Tc-labelled monoclonal antibody raised against white cells, can also be used.

2. Uptake of labelled white cells is seen in the liver, spleen and marrow, which is normal. There is curvilinear abnormal activity clearly seen in the right breast. This is due to infection after a breast augmentation operation, which was the cause of the fever.

3. A chest X-ray will show the presence of the breast prostheses.

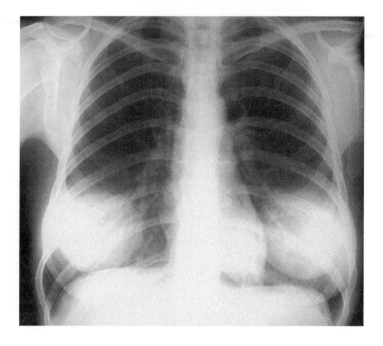

TEACHING POINT

- Not all chest pain is cardiac or pulmonary in origin, and a careful history is vital, especially where there may have been previous surgery.

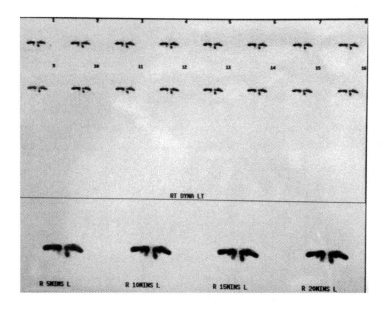

RT DYNR LT

R 5MINS L   R 10MINS L   R 15MINS L   R 20MINS L

1. What is this examination and how is it performed?
2. What does it show?
3. In which clinical condition is it used?
4. What examination would you do next?

ANSWERS

1. A lacrimal drainage study. One drop of ^{99m}Tc pertechnetate is instilled in each eye, and a dynamic acquisition of 16 10-s frames obtained, followed by four 5-min frames over 20 min.
2. Bilateral block to drainage.
3. Epiphora.
4. A radiological dacrocystogram may also be performed.

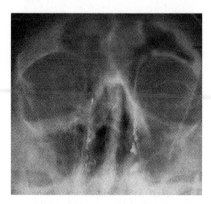

This shows the contrast held up in the nasolacrimal ducts. A pair of normal studies are shown below for comparison.

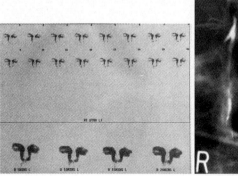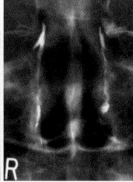

TEACHING POINTS

- The radiological study requires injection of contrast under pressure, and so will show the anatomy, but in the isotope study, the pertechnetate is given as a drop into each eye. The drainage is therefore physiological and gives information as to how the lacrimal drainage system is functioning and will demonstrate the level of block. This is important for the surgical management of epiphora.
- Isotope studies are marginally more sensitive and have the additional advantage of being more acceptable to the patient.

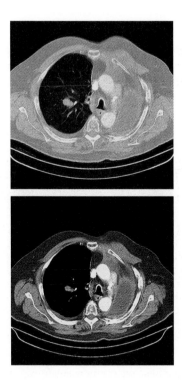

This patient had previously had a left pneumonectomy for a carcinoma. On the follow-up CT some years later, a solid lesion was shown in the right mid-zone. The clinical problem was how to investigate this further.

1. What would you suggest?

ANSWER

1. A biopsy is not indicated as the lesion is too deep and the patient would probably not tolerate a pneumothorax. The next investigation was a PET scan using ^{18}FDG.

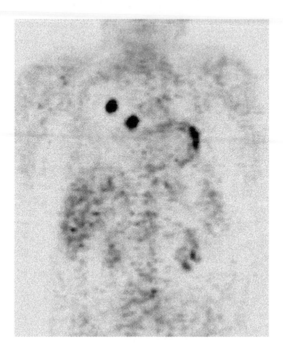

This shows intense uptake in the peripheral lesion seen on the CT images, but there is also activity at the right hilum. These findings are indicative of a second primary lung tumour with hilar nodal deposits not well shown on the CT. In view of the previous left pneumonectomy, chemotherapy is the only option.

TEACHING POINTS

- The positron-emitting isotope is ^{18}F as ^{18}FDG. ^{18}FDG is a glucose analogue that undergoes phosphorylation to ^{18}FDG-6-P, but then stays in the cell and does not take any further part in glycolysis. It is used because, in general, malignant cells overexpress GLUT transporter receptors and thus take up ^{18}FDG avidly. ^{18}FDG can be used to study many tumours that have an increased metabolic need.
- Lung cancer is common and increasing, and constitutes 22% of all cancers in men and 8% in women. T1N0M0 and T2N0M0 non-small cell tumours are curable by surgery, so early diagnosis is crucial.
- Primary diagnosis of lung cancer is usually made by biopsy following more conventional imaging, such as CT or MRI. The role of PET is in

the staging of potentially operable disease (hence, although both small cell and non-small cell carcinomas take up tracer, it is usually only used in the latter); in follow-up; and in cases of suspected recurrence. It has an important role if there is the suspicion of adrenal secondaries; if the adrenals take up [18]FDG there is a strong possibility of malignant disease.

- Approximately 15% of patients have distant disease which is not suspected and overall about 30% of patients have changes in management as a result of the PET scan.

- In recurrent disease PET scanning is more sensitive than CT because surgery and radiotherapy distort the anatomy. In looking at recurrent disease, it is important to wait until any inflammatory changes related to the treatment modality have subsided. For chemotherapy this is 2–3 weeks, for surgery 6 weeks and for radiotherapy 3 months. All surgical sites will take up tracer until fully healed.

- Adriamycin reduces FDG activity and so if it has been given, false negative PET scans could arise.

- In normal cases, activity is seen in the base of the brain (although the brain is usually excluded from the field of view) and heart, and some may well be seen in the salivary glands and pharyngeal muscles.

- A word of caution: if the patient is tense, there may well be increased uptake in the neck muscles due to their increased activity, and similarly, if the patient talks a lot during the post-injection phase, then there will be significant uptake in the larynx.

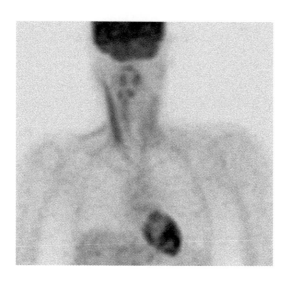

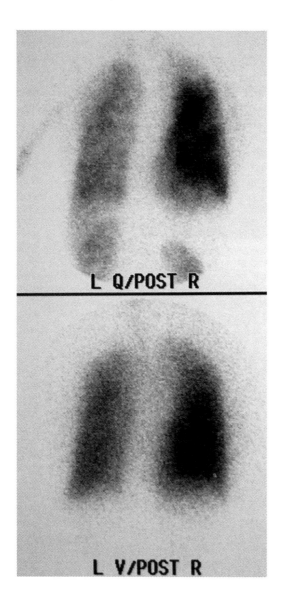

L Q/POST R

L V/POST R

1. What does this lung scan show and is it normal?

ANSWER

1. Whilst the perfusion scan is slightly patchy, there are no obvious defects. The ventilation scan is normal and there is no evidence of pulmonary emboli on these posterior views. However, activity in the kidneys is seen on the perfusion scan and this is abnormal.

This activity indicates that there must be a right-to-left shunt, as otherwise the ^{99m}Tc-labelled microspheres could not access the systemic circulation. Imaging the head can demonstrate the presence of the shunt.

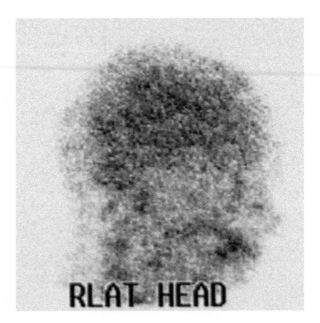

An alternative explanation would be the presence of free pertechnetate, but this is discounted in this case as there is no uptake in the thyroid or gastric mucosa.

TEACHING POINTS

- It is crucial that the requesting clinician informs the Nuclear Medicine department that the patient has a shunt, and in fact this is a legal requirement under Ionising Radiation (Medical Exposure) Regulations [IR(ME)R].
- If microspheres enter the cerebral circulation, there is a theoretical risk of small strokes. Reducing the number of microspheres per ml injected can lessen this danger, and freshly prepared microspheres should be used to lessen the potential of them clumping.
- Although a right-to-left shunt is a relative contraindication for a lung scan, remember that, historically, microspheres were used to measure blood flow to kidneys and brain.

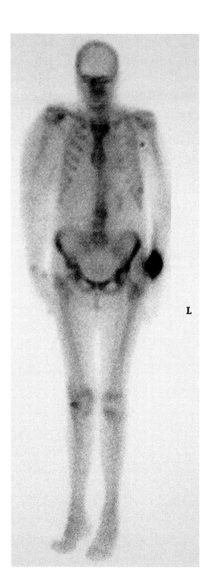

1. What does this image show?

ANSWER

1. Intense activity in the dorsum of the left hand and activity in the left axilla. This is a tissued injection with axillary nodal uptake.

TEACHING POINTS

- Tissuing can be avoided by selecting larger veins for injection and not using the dorsum of the hand. It is important not to inject tracer on the side where there is known or suspected pathology. It may be necessary to use the veins in the feet in some patients.
- Axillary nodal uptake can also be seen in metastatic disease, but in this case is due to lymphatic drainage from isotope in the soft tissues of the hand. This is the principle of lymphatic drainage used in sentinal node imaging, where the isotope is deliberately injected intradermally or intra-tumourally.

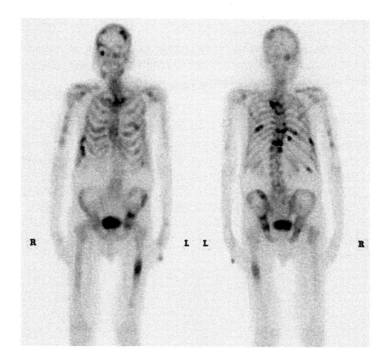

This patient presented with generalized pains. This is the bone scan.

1. What does it show?

ANSWER

1. Multiple areas of abnormally increased uptake, scattered throughout the central skeleton and upper left femur. This distribution of abnormal activity is due to widespread metastatic disease.

TEACHING POINTS

- In cases such as this, there is no real problem with the diagnosis, but whilst the bone scan is very sensitive to alteration in bone metabolism, it is not specific for the site of the primary lesion. There may be clues on the scan, such as an absent kidney or a large prostatic impression in the base of the bladder with the patient catheterised, as below.

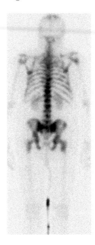

- In cases where there is only one area of abnormal activity, further correlative imaging, usually MRI or CT, may be needed.
- It is usually fairly easy to differentiate metastases from fractures, which appear punctate and often in a linear manner, as below, in the ribs. Vertebral collapse appears as a plate-like area of increased uptake (below left), and osteoarthritis is usually associated with the inner aspect of the curve and is due to uptake in osteophytes (below right).

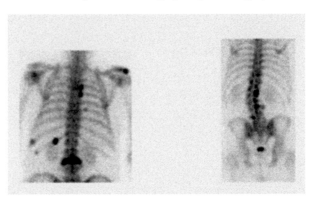

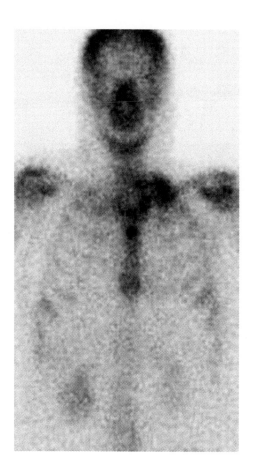

1. What can be seen on this bone scan?
2. What is the differential diagnosis?

ANSWERS

1. An area of markedly increased uptake at the left apex, in the region of the first rib.
2. A metastasis, Paget's disease or a bone neoplasm, as trauma to this site is most unusual.

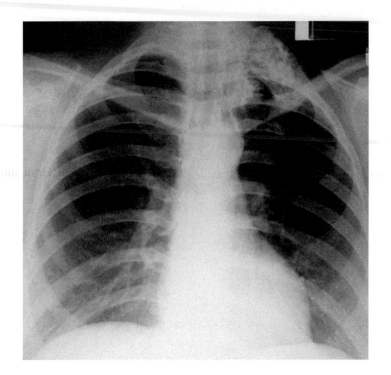

The above chest X-ray shows the grossly abnormal left first rib, which is expanded and has irregular calcification within it. The appearance is that of an enchondroma, a benign bone neoplasm.

TEACHING POINTS

- Bone scanning is very sensitive in the detection of metabolic abnormalities, but it has a poor specificity. When the bone scan is combined with an X-ray, the high sensitivity of the bone scan is complemented by the high specificity of the X-ray. It is impossible to make the diagnosis from the bone scan alone.
- The uptake in the region of the sternomanubrial joint is a normal variant. However, in patients with breast cancer it may indicate a solitary bone metastasis.
- In patients with chondromata, the role of bone scanning is to provide a whole body skeletal survey.

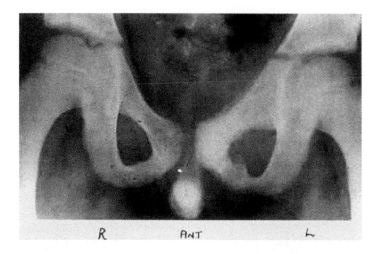

R   ANT   L

This young boy complained of pain in the left side of his pelvis of short duration, and fever. No other history was available. An X-ray of the pelvis was obtained.

1. What can you see?
2. What is the differential diagnosis?
3. What would you do next?

ANSWERS

1. An area of increased bone density in the left superior pubic ramus contained by the unfused epiphyses. The bone texture is abnormal and irregular, showing patchy bone destruction with well-defined periosteal new bone clearly visible. A soft tissue mass is seen lying superior to the bone.
2. Infection or tumour.
3. Further imaging is needed urgently.

A bone scan (below) showed diffusely increased uptake in the affected bone and bladder displacement. This displacement is caused by the soft tissue mass, which would be well demonstrated on CT or MRI. These appearances suggest bone neoplasm, and in this position and age group the likeliest diagnosis is Ewing's sarcoma. Biopsy is needed to confirm the diagnosis and remember to send a specimen for microbiology to exclude infection.

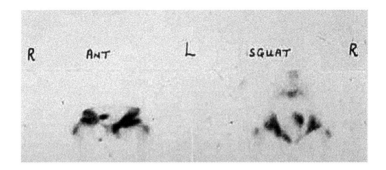

TEACHING POINTS

- In children, always consider infection *and* primary bone neoplasm, as their appearances can be very similar.
- In Ewing's sarcoma, CT or MRI show the soft tissue component and the resulting distortion, as well as the abnormal bone. CT of the chest should also be performed as these tumours metastasize to the lungs early.

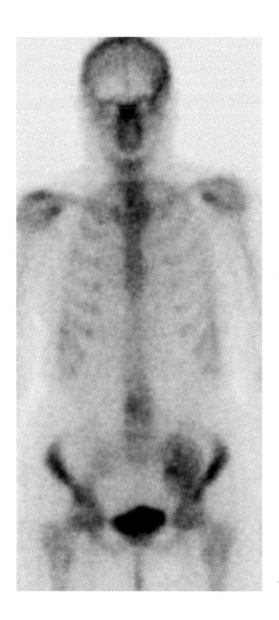

1. What can you see on this scan?

ANSWER

1. No obvious abnormalities are seen in the skeleton, which is normal. However, the kidneys are not in their normal position and there is an area of abnormal, reniform uptake in the left iliac fossa, overlying the iliac wing. This is a renal transplant.

This is confirmed on an intravenous urogram (below), which shows the left iliac fossa kidney clearly, although caution should be taken with potentially nephrotoxic contrast media in transplants. Ultrasound can also be used to monitor the state of the transplant, particularly colour duplex scanning showing renal blood flow.

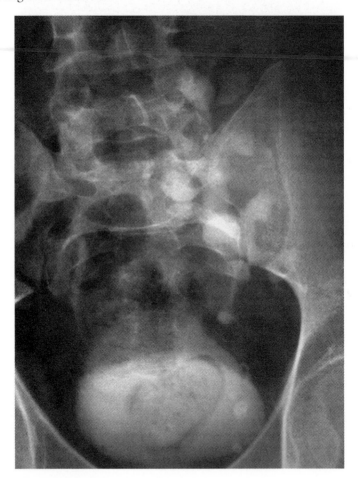

TEACHING POINTS

- Transplanted kidneys can be in either iliac fossa and are often not mentioned on the request form. Ensure that there are no normally situated kidneys.
- In renal failure, isotope scans have a high background, giving very poor images. In this case, the images are normal, and there is no renal failure.

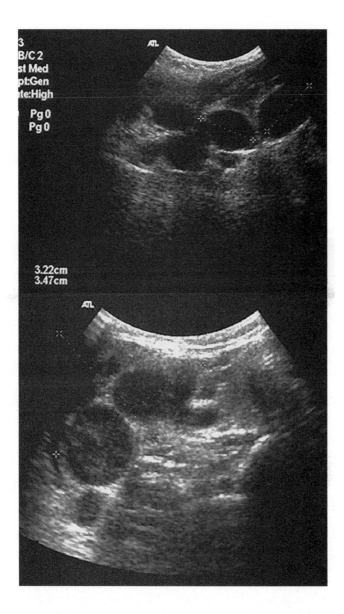

This young patient presented with a lump in the right side of the neck.

1. What do these images show?

ANSWER

1. Large inhomogeneous nodes in the neck which are highly suggestive of a lymphoma.

To confirm the diagnosis, a biopsy was performed, and to stage the disease a PET scan was carried out using ^{18}FDG.

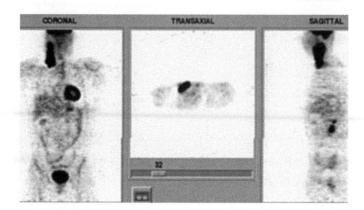

These images show the intense activity in the nodal mass in the right side of the neck, but more importantly also show that there are no other foci of increased activity. Note that ^{18}FDG is also seen in the heart and brain, and as it is excreted via the kidneys, it is seen in the bladder. Occasionally, as here, some gut activity is also seen.

TEACHING POINTS

- ^{18}FDG-PET imaging is widely used in the staging of many tumours. The images must be read in conjunction with other imaging modalities, mainly CT. This allows the differentiation of tumour activity and post-therapy fibrosis. The modern generations of PET scanners incorporate a CT scanner and thus sequential PET/CT scans are acquired allowing co-registration of any abnormalities.
- Not all lymphomas take up FDG. Hodgkin's disease and high-grade non-Hodgkin lymphoma take it up avidly, but low grade poorly. There is increasing use of ^{18}FDG-PET in lymphoma assessment, not only in the initial staging but also in assessing the response to treatment and relapse. The management changes in about 30% of cases as a result of PET staging.

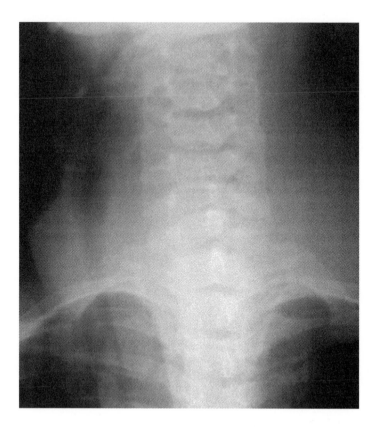

This patient suffered from dysphagia and was sent for this X-ray by the GP.

1. What does the X-ray show?
2. What is your diagnosis?
3. What else could you do?

ANSWERS

1. Significant tracheal deviation to the right, with a large soft–tissue mass centrally.
2. A large goitre.
3. A radionuclide scan.

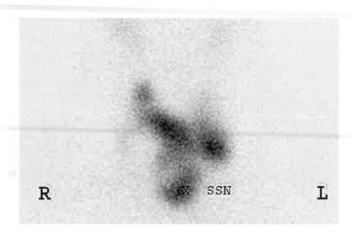

This scan shows a large inhomogeneous thyroid, with some retrosternal extension. This is typical of a multinodular goitre. This condition can also be shown on ultrasound.

TEACHING POINTS

- If no nodules are palpable, and the thyroid function tests are normal, there is no indication to image the thyroid either with ultrasound or nuclear medicine. Screening of the neck is useless without clinical indications of disease. In cases where a multinodular goitre is suspected, nuclear medicine images will give more useful information but need to be justified under IR(ME)R since in many cases the ultrasound will identify multiple nodules. A pertechnetate scan may be used to confirm the mass is thyroid. It is also important for the surgeon to know if there is retrosternal extension and this is best seen on a nuclear medicine scan. If there is a reason to suspect malignancy then the pertechnetate scan may be helpful to identify which nodules are cold and thus should be sampled rather than those which are functioning.
- The radionuclide scan is of use when there is a dominant nodule and there is a question of functioning. A functioning nodule can be considered benign since malignancy is extremely uncommon.
- Where the goitre causes tracheal displacement, stridor can be a problem. This can be made worse if there is bleeding into a cystic nodule.
- Usually, thyroid radionuclide imaging uses ^{99m}Tc as pertechnetate. In cases of a significant retrosternal goitre, ^{123}I may be used since it gives a clearer image, but in practice ^{99m}Tc often gives enough detail for clinical purposes.

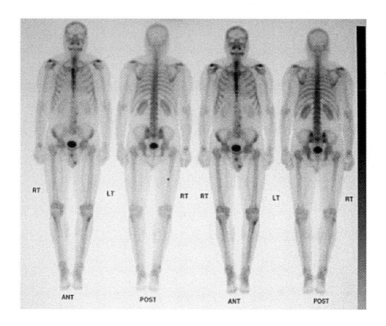

1. What two abnormalities does this image show?
2. What is the tracer used and what is the diagnostic reference level (DRL)?
3. Why are there two sets of images?

ANSWERS

1. (i) Increased uptake in the sternum. This is linear and is typical of that seen in a sternotomy wound. (ii) A focus of uptake in the right mid-femur on the posterior view on the left-hand set of images. This is not seen on any of the other views and thus is an artefact caused by a spot of paint on the viewing box.
2. A diphosphonate labelled with ^{99m}Tc. The DRL is set individually by each department. Many use the levels set by ARSAC.
3. There are usually two sets of images because in order to view the axial skeleton the image intensity needs to be less than that when viewing the peripheral skeleton.

TEACHING POINTS

- It can take up to 1 year for the increased uptake in a bone fracture to return to normal.
- Always check other views to ensure any abnormality seen is on all appropriate views.
- All exposures in nuclear medicine and radiology have to be within the departmental DRL. It is, however, permitted to alter the exposure if circumstances indicate that the usual activity given will not result in a diagnostic scan. For example, in patients who are considerably overweight it may be necessary to increase the activity given. Also, if a patient is in pain and unable to lie still for long enough it may be appropriate to increase the activity given and reduce the time taken for the scan.

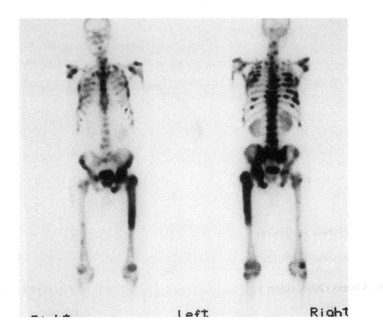

Left   Right

1. What does this image show?

ANSWER

1. A bone scan showing intense uptake in the left hemi-pelvis and upper half of the left femur, which is typical of Paget's disease. However, there are also multiple areas of irregular increased uptake within the ribs, and these are not due to Paget's disease, but to secondary deposits.

Paget's normally affects long bones and starts at the articular surface, as below in the right tibia. When it affects the ribs, the uptake is much more along the rib and the rib appears enlarged.

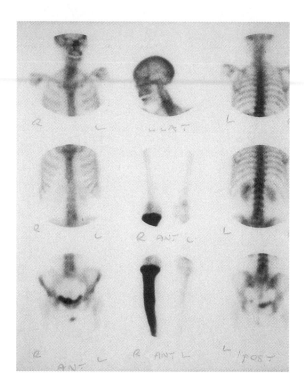

TEACHING POINT

- Paget's and secondaries may co-exist, but obviously it is impossible on a bone scan to see whether there is a secondary within an area of Paget's.

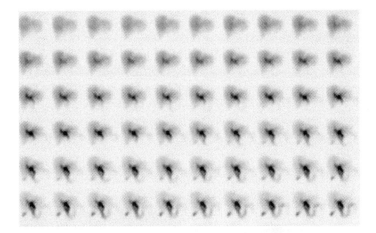

This is a series of images in a dynamic study.

1. What is the study?
2. What is the tracer used?
3. What abnormality is this study used to show?

ANSWERS

1. A normal hepatobiliary scan.
2. A variety of tracers are available but they are all iminodiacetates labelled with ^{99m}Tc.
3. These scans may be used in the diagnosis of acute cholecystitis. If there is gallbladder uptake, then this excludes acute cholecystitis. The absence of uptake in the gallbladder indicates gallbladder dysfunction. These scans are also used to detect biliary leaks, biliary obstruction and, in liver transplanatation, to evaluate allograft function.

Ultrasound is now more widely used for gallstone disease.

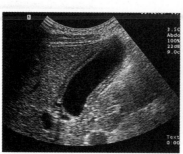 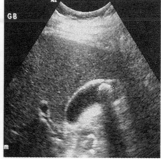

TEACHING POINT

- HIDA scans are now mainly used to investigate post-surgical leaks.

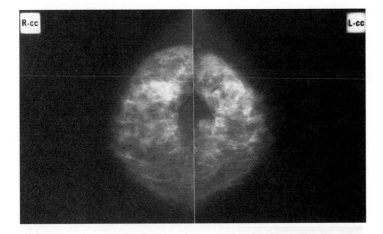

This patient with a strong family history of breast cancer attended for a mammogram.

1. As the mammogram was equivocal, what supplementary investigations could be performed?

ANSWER

1. Breasts can be further evaluated by ultrasound, scintimammography or MRI.

Scintimammography (below) is carried out using sestamibi, a tumour-seeking ^{99m}Tc-labelled agent. It is most useful in dense breasts, or post-operative or post-DXR cases where the mammogram is difficult to interpret.

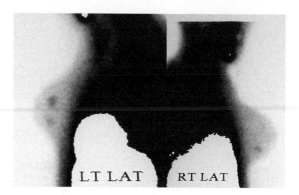

These images show foci of increased uptake in both breasts, making the diagnosis of bilateral carcinoma of the breasts. There is no axillary nodal activity, although this is rarely seen. Normal breasts show a very even activity with no foci, as below.

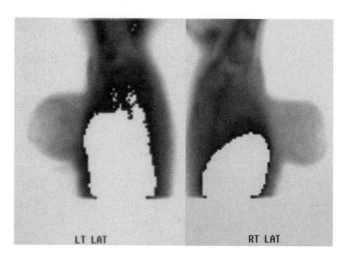

TEACHING POINT

- The sestamibi must be injected into the dorsum of the foot, so that if there is extravasation of activity, it is trapped in the iliac nodes. If the activity is injected in the arm, activity may be seen in the axilla, and it would not be possible to differentiate a malignant node from the result of extravasation of activity.

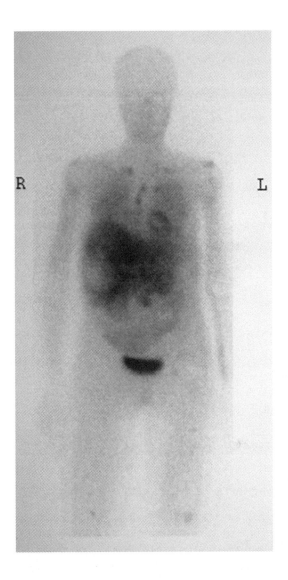

1. What is this examination?
2. What does it show?
3. What examination would you do next and what else might you consider?

ANSWERS

1. An ^{111}In-octreotide scan. The normal distribution is in liver, spleen, bowel and urinary tract. Activity elsewhere is pathological.
2. This scan shows obvious hepatomegaly, with a large 'cold' area in the right lobe, and also several areas of increased uptake in the lungs and mediastinum, and in several bones. These are metastatic carcinoid deposits.
3. A CT and a representative example from the abdomen is shown below. This shows the multiple hepatic deposits and can guide biopsy, particularly should only one lesion be seen on the octreotide image.

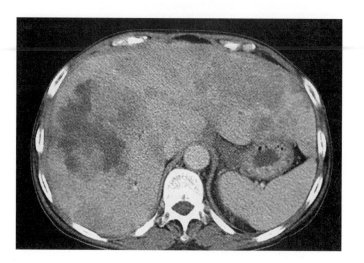

TEACHING POINTS

- An octreotide scan can be differentiated from a gallium scan because in the latter there is no bowel uptake. If the tracer were MIBG, uptake in the parotid glands would be expected.
- Octreotide scans are used to show neuroendocrine tumours, such as carcinoid, neuroblastoma, medullary cell thyroid carcinoma, phaeochromocytoma, gastrinoma, etc.
- Patients should also have an ^{123}I–MIBG scan to identify additional lesions and assess the feasibility of tracer therapy with ^{131}I–MIBG. Some lesions are shown with one tracer but not with the other. Octreotide imaging is more sensitive than ^{123}I–MIBG for the detection of lesions. Octreotide can also be labelled with ^{90}Y, a β-emitter, for therapy.
- SPECT should also be undertaken to delineate the deposits more effectively.

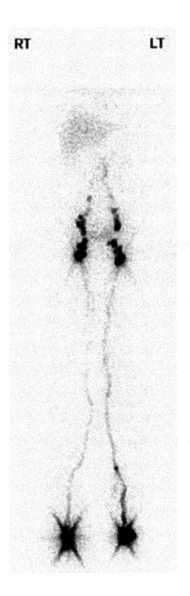

This patient presented with swollen legs.

1. What is this investigation?
2. What does it show?

ANSWERS

1. A lymphoscintigram. This is performed by injecting a small dose of ^{99m}Tc-labelled colloid into the first web space of each foot, and imaging sequentially to show the clearance of the colloid by the lymphatic system.
2. Clearance is usually fairly rapid and symmetrical, reaching the iliac nodes by 2 h. Delay is suggestive of stasis, e.g. Milroy's disease.

There may be one or more main lymphatic pathways and activity should also be seen in the liver. Occasionally, leakage into the soft tissues of the calf occurs in cases of lymphatic insufficiency, as below, where there is some leakage of activity into the soft tissues around the right ankle.

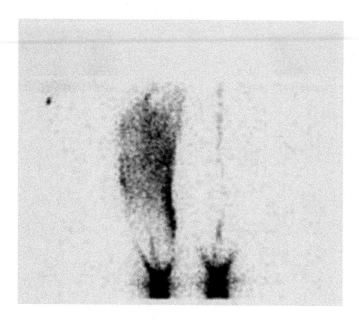

TEACHING POINT

● The lymphoscintigram is easy to perform and may be quantitated. It is very useful in evaluating patients with swollen legs, where there is no obvious vascular cause. It obviates the need for a radiographic lymphogram. This has been described by Burnand KG, McGuinness CL, Lagattolla NRF, Browse NL, El-Aradi A, Nunan T. Value of isotope lymphography in the diagnosis of lymphoedema of the leg. *Br J Surg* 2002; **89**: 74.

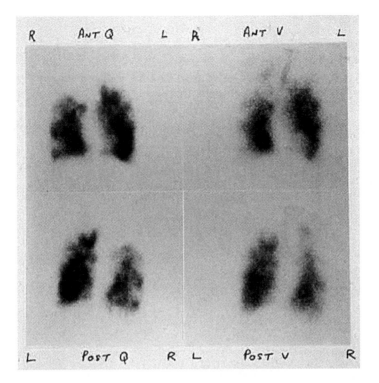

This child had a persistent cough and failed to grow well.

1. What does this lung scan show?
2. What further investigation is needed?

ANSWERS

1. Patchy distribution of activity in both the ventilation and perfusion images, with no obvious perfusion mismatches, and matched defects in the right upper lobe. In fact, the ventilation images appear worse. These appearances suggest widespread parenchymal disease, with widespread infection.
2. A chest X-ray.

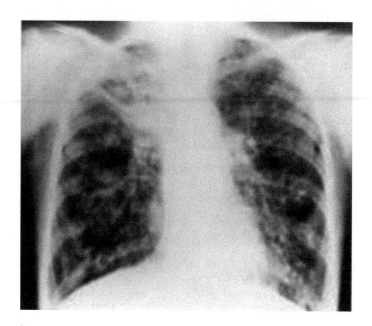

This chest X-ray shows loss of volume of the right upper lobe and multiple cystic areas within both lungs, some showing consolidation. The patient is also very thin. The appearances are those of cystic fibrosis with areas of infection and a probable mucous plug in the right upper lobe bronchus.

TEACHING POINTS

- As in adult practice, a current chest X-ray must always be available when reporting paediatric lung scans.
- Further biochemical tests will confirm the diagnosis of cystic fibrosis, as will a high-resolution CT scan.
- Nowadays, a V/Q scan is unlikely to be performed in patients with parenchymal disease.

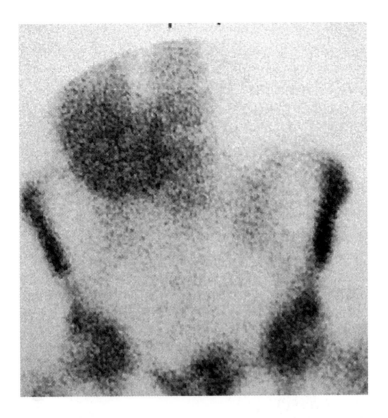

1. What does this bone scan show?

ANSWER

1. A large reniform area of increased uptake lying to the right of the mid-line, and no evidence of any renal activity on the left.

These are the appearances of renal crossed fused ectopia. A transplant is unlikely given the shape and position. The crossed fused ectopia can be clearly shown on an intravenous urogram (below).

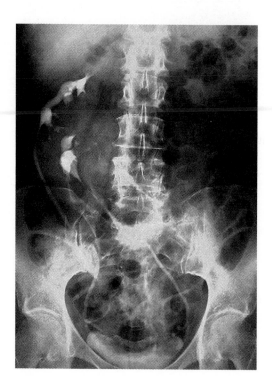

TEACHING POINTS

- Crossed fused ectopia only occurs on the right and is of no real significance to the patient. It is occasionally diagnosed on a bone scan, as here, performed for other reasons.
- It is important in all renal studies of ectopic kidneys to acquire anterior images. The differential function can be more difficult to calculate accurately since there is variable attenuation caused by the pelvic bones.

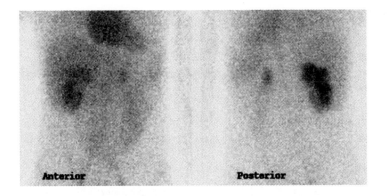

This patient had this investigation as part of their work-up.

1. What is this investigation?
2. What does it show and is it normal?

ANSWERS

1. Activity is seen widely distributed throughout the blood pool, heart, liver, spleen and kidneys. The images give no clue as to the type of scan – it could be an early set of images from a dynamic renal scan (MAG3 or DTPA), a DMSA scan or even an early blood-pool phase of a bone scan. The scan is in fact a DMSA scan, used to show where there is functioning renal tissue.

2. The patient is in chronic renal failure with a creatinine level of 1323 μmol/L. In addition, the left kidney is small and scarred and there is obvious scarring in the right kidney, which is of normal size.

A normal DMSA scan (below) has very little background activity.

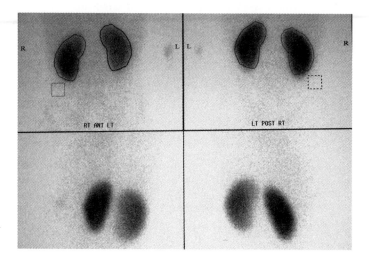

TEACHING POINTS

- Normally, DMSA images are obtained 3 h after injection, but in cases of chronic renal failure, it may be necessary to image as late as 6 h after injection.
- DMSA is taken up by the proximal tubular cells in the renal cortex and identifies functioning renal tissue. The most common use is the evaluation of scarring in children's kidneys following UTIs, and to follow up renal function in cases of impaired renal function. They are not dynamic scans.
- The differential function is accurate in normal renal function to about ±7%. In renal failure this accuracy is less and so should be interpreted with caution.

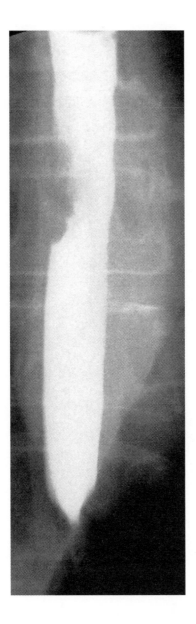

This patient presented with mild difficulty in swallowing and occasional central chest pain.

1. What is this investigation?
2. What does it show?

ANSWERS

1. A barium swallow.
2. Mucosal irregularity in the wall of the oesophagus. The diagnosis is carcinoma of the oesophagus.

Apart from biopsy proof, the disease needs to be staged, and this can be done using CT or PET. Below is a PET image of carcinoma of the oesophagus.

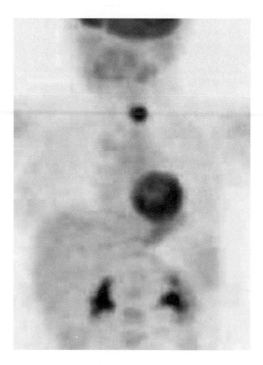

The intense uptake can be seen in the mid-oesophagus at the tumour site, but more importantly there is no abnormal uptake at the hila, in the liver or abdomen.

TEACHING POINTS

- This scan shows physiological uptake of FDG in the brain, heart and renal tract.
- It is important prior to surgery to be sure there are no distant metastases.
- Staging should include PET where available, as PET indicates the metabolic activity of lesions seen on CT and MRI, and this is relevant to treatment. A review of the literature showed an estimated 20% change in management based on the PET scan. PET cannot be expected to identify local lymph node involvement. Endoscopic ultrasound is used for local staging.

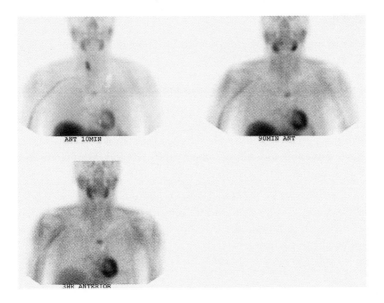

1. What type of scan is this and what isotope is used?
2. What does this series of images show?
3. How is the scan performed?

ANSWERS

1. A scan to image a parathyroid adenoma. The radiopharmaceutical used is ^{99m}Tc–labelled sestamibi.
2. There has been a partial thyroidectomy on the left and there is a focus of activity persisting in the left aorto-pulmonary window. This represents an ectopic parathyroid. Surgery to remove ectopic parathyroids in this position can be extremely difficult.
3. There are a variety of protocols. The scan shown is performed by injecting the sestamibi, and taking images at 10, 20 and 90 min, and possibly also at 4 h.

Sestamibi is taken up by the thyroid and parathyroids, but is washed out of normal tissue much faster than out of tumours. Thus, parathyroid adenomas can be detected, although there is no way of differentiating between a carcinoma and an adenoma.

Below is a left lower parathyroid adenoma, with activity persisting at 4 h.

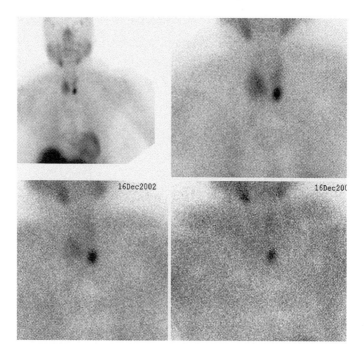

Normal parathyroids, and hyperplastic glands, are not seen on these images.

TEACHING POINT

- The first image must include the whole thorax; later ones can focus on the neck if nothing is seen in the thorax. As there is increasing use of keyhole day surgery, accurate pre-operative localization is important.

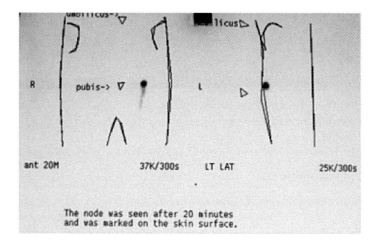

ant 20M   37K/300s   LT LAT   25K/300s

The node was seen after 20 minutes
and was marked on the skin surface.

1. What is this study?
2. What does it show?
3. What is the clinical indication?
4. What other imaging technique accompanies this scan?

ANSWERS

1. A sentinel node study in a patient with a malignant melanoma. The area around the excised melanoma is injected with ^{99m}Tc-labelled nanocolloid, which is taken up in the lymphatics.
2. A focus of increased uptake in the left inguinal region.
3. Patients with intermediate Breslow thickness melanomas (1–4 mm).
4. Intraoperative probe and methylene blue injection is also used to localize the sentinel node.

TEACHING POINTS

- In cases with thin melanomas, the likelihood of spread is very low and thus the test is of little use for screening. Local excision is all that is required. In thick (>4 mm) tumours, the likelihood of spread is high and thus imaging to look for distant metastases is needed.
- Sentinel node scanning is the most sensitive way of identifying the lymphatic drainage of melanomas. There are an average of 2.7 nodes per patient and in up to 34% of patients, drainage is noted outside the expected area. The scan below shows a sentinel node study from a patient with a melanoma in the middle of the back. The region of the injection is masked so that the much lower activity in the sentinel nodes is easily seen. Four sentinel nodes are seen, two in each axilla.

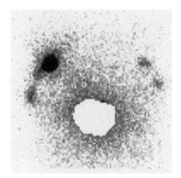

- Sentinel node studies are also performed in cases of breast carcinoma, with the nanocolloid being injected into the tumour, and the patient scanned some 3 h later. This will identify the sentinel node(s) prior to surgery.

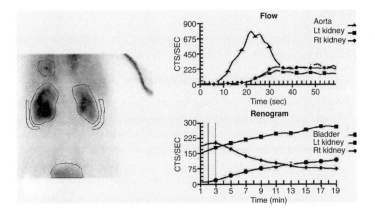

1. What is this investigation?
2. What does it show?
3. What pharmacological interventions can be performed in renography?
4. What special preparations are required in renography?

ANSWERS

1. A MAG3 dynamic renogram, labelled with ^{99m}Tc. The indication was a patient who presented with left renal pain and the ultrasound showed a full collecting system on the left, suggesting a degree of obstruction.
2. This scan is abnormal. It shows, on the left, the summed view with the regions of interest drawn around the kidneys, background, heart and bladder. The computer then generates two sets of background corrected curves, on the right. The upper set shows the clearance through the heart and into the kidneys. There is symmetrical inflow of isotope into the kidneys. The lower graph shows the uptake and clearance of isotope and there is normal clearance on the right but a continuously rising curve on the left.
3. Furosemide takes about 15 min to produce a maximum diuresis. Thus, it may be given prior to injection of tracer in order that the diuresis is occurring throughout the whole of the renogram. If it is given at the end of the renogram and a further 10 min of acquisition is made, the furosemide will only just be beginning to act when the study ends.
4. Patients must be well hydrated prior to the study.

The image below from an intravenous urogram series shows normal excretion on the right, and a dilated collecting system and persisting nephrogram on the left, which is typical of obstruction.

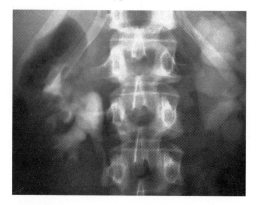

TEACHING POINTS

- Whilst the IVU gives the anatomy, the dynamic renogram gives the physiology and function.
- It is good practice to measure the urine volume during the study by asking the patient to void prior to the scan and again after. By knowing the time interval, the urinary flow rate can be calculated, which lends confidence to the interpretation of the renogram if the curves are abnormal.
- A final post void image may help in cases where the appearances suggest obstruction with the patient lying down, but the renal tracts empty when the patient stands up, or the renal tracts fail to empty due to a full bladder.
- Renal impairment or very dilated outflow tracts can give poor clearance of tracer and a late image an hour or more after the injection of tracer may be useful.

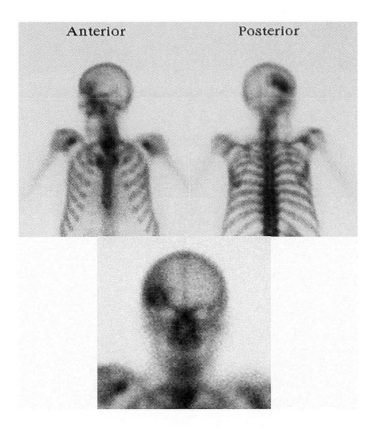

These are views of the skull and thorax from a bone scan.

1. What do they show?
2. What imaging would you do next?

ANSWERS

1. Abnormal activity is clearly seen in the right parietal area. This could be due to fibrous dysplasia, a sphenoid wing meningioma, or anything that alters the blood–brain barrier.
2. A CT head scan.

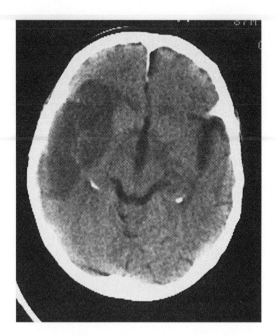

This shows a low attenuation area in the right middle cerebral artery territory, typical of a cerebrovascular accident. As the blood–brain barrier is breached, bone agent can enter the brain and so give the appearances shown on the bone scan.

TEACHING POINT

● Although bone scans primarily show the skeleton, remember that bone agent will also show lesions in the kidneys, such as cysts or tumours, which are shown as photon-deficient areas within the kidney. Soft tissue lesions such as lipomata are occasionally seen, and when the blood–brain barrier is breached activity is seen within the brain, as in this case. (A more exhaustive list is given on p 32.)

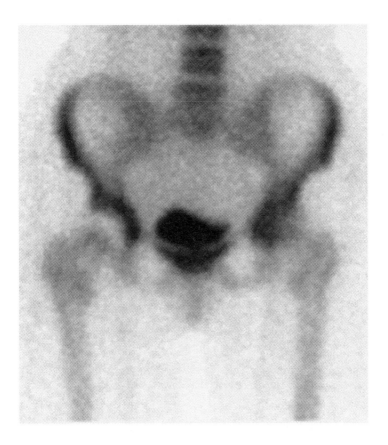

This patient was referred for a bone scan with a history of recent right hip pain. No other information was given.

1. What does the scan show?
2. What is your diagnosis?
3. What else would be helpful?

ANSWERS

1. An obvious area of photopenia in the region of the right femoral capital epiphysis.
2. In view of the history, the suspicion of aseptic necrosis must be raised.
3. However, as the patient said that she had had an operation on her hip (type unknown) an X-ray should be obtained.

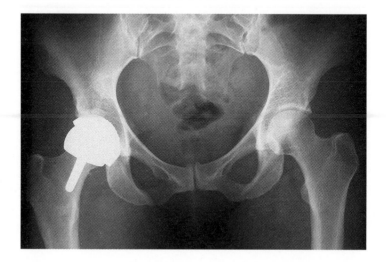

The image above shows a mini–THR on the right and is the obvious cause of the photopenic area. No other lesions are seen and there are no abnormal areas of uptake on the bone scan to suggest loosening or infection.

TEACHING POINT

- The request form was incomplete and inaccurate and as such does not comply with IR(ME)R regulations. These make it clear that it is the referrer's responsibility to ensure the relevant clinical information is on the request form. However, they also state the person justifying the clinical exposure must have the results of other imaging procedures available.

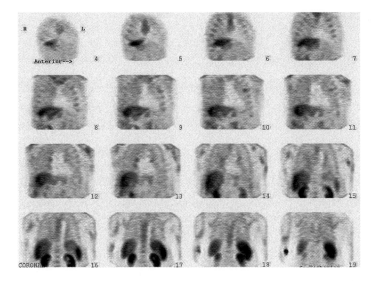

1. What is this investigation and what does it demonstrate?
2. What can be seen?

ANSWERS

1. A tomographic study of the thorax, using a ^{99m}Tc-labelled somatostatin receptor, called depreotide. This labels the somatostatin receptors, typically types 1 and 2, which are overexpressed in tumours, and is specifically aimed at demonstrating lung cancer.
2. The lesion can be clearly seen in the left upper lobe (slice 10), but there is also abnormal activity seen in both hila (slice 13), indicating that the tumour has metastasized.

TEACHING POINTS

- The advantage of this imaging compound is that it is ^{99m}Tc based, and so can be used to image lung cancer on any gamma-camera capable of SPECT, unlike PET which needs a dedicated PET camera. The image below (from another patient), using ^{18}FDG, is of a lung cancer in the right upper lobe and shows the tumour clearly and also that there are no deposits.

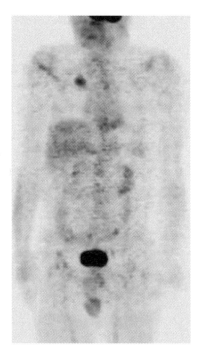

- Both depreotide images and PET show metabolically active lesions, and so differentiate scars from tumour, both of which may look very similar on a chest X-ray or CT. Depreotide is sensitive but not specific, so histology is always required to confirm the diagnosis.

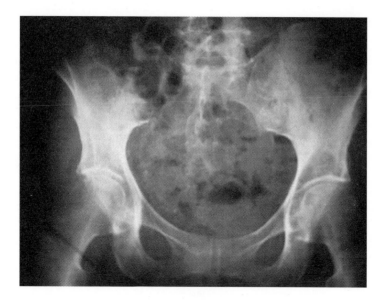

This patient presented to A&E with back pain, mainly on the right. The above pelvic X-ray was taken.

1. What can you say about it?
2. What other investigations would you consider?

ANSWERS

1. There is a large defect in the right sacrum, but it is extremely difficult to see this on conventional X-rays because there is a significant amount of overlying bowel gas. The only clue on the plain film is that the lower margin of the sacrum is not seen.
2. The best way of looking for bone pathology is bone scanning, since this will demonstrate any focal pathology and is not hindered by overlying bowel gas.

The bone scan below clearly demonstrates the extent of the right sacral lesion.

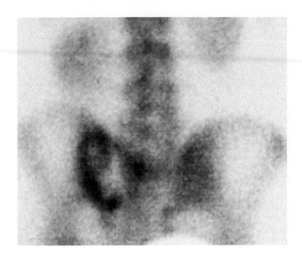

TEACHING POINTS

- Bone scans are extremely sensitive at showing altered bone metabolism, but are not specific for pathology. In malignant bone disease what is being imaged is the bony response to the tumour, not the malignant focus itself. This accounts for the fact that lytic lesions tend not to be seen on bone scans but sclerotic lesions do. Rapidly growing lesions may not be detected on a bone scan because the tumour is growing so fast that the bone around it is unable to mount a response.
- In the pelvis, bladder activity may obscure the sacrum. It is then necessary either to perform a squat view (below) or to acquire a local view at 24 h; the latter takes a significant time although it does not affect the rest of the departmental workload. This typical squat view shows the separation of the bladder from the sacrum.

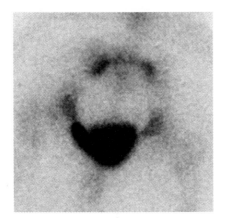

- Other special views often used are oblique or lateral views of the chest to identify rib lesions, or an 'arms up' view to move the scapulae away from the ribs to see if a focus of uptake is due to the tip of the scapula over-lying a rib.
- To obtain the final diagnosis in this case, biopsy would be needed. CT and MRI are also good at showing the bone destruction.

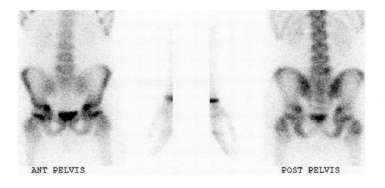

ANT PELVIS   POST PELVIS

This young ballerina presented with low back pain. The plain X-rays are normal.

1. What does this image show?

ANSWER

1. The ^{99m}Tc–MDP planar bone scan shows minimally increased uptake in the right pedicle of L5, but no firm diagnosis could be made from this study. Note that the scan is of a young person, with unfused epiphyses, which are clearly seen as areas of increased uptake in the femoral neck, acetabulum and wrist.

A tomographic study was also carried out (below). This is known as SPECT (single photon emission CT), which is the nuclear medicine version of conventional CT. The data is acquired with the camera heads rotating around the patient, and then reconstituted in sagittal, coronal and transverse planes.

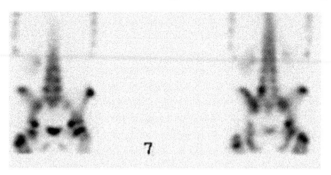

These coronal images clearly show that there is abnormal uptake in the right pedicle and the likeliest diagnosis is a pars fracture. This was confirmed on MRI; the fracture is identified by the white oedema just below the bone of the pars. A normal pars with no fracture is seen at the same level above.

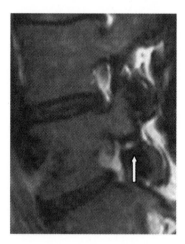

TEACHING POINT

- Low back pain in young patients with immature skeletons is almost always due to trauma, although the differential diagnosis must include a spinal osteoid osteoma or malignancy. Usually, a careful history will elicit the trauma.

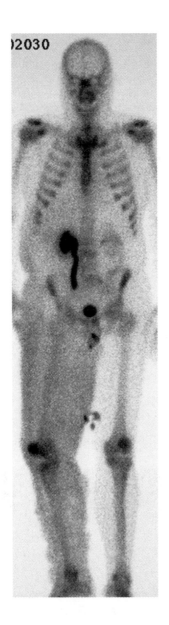

02030

This patient with melanoma was sent for a bone scan.

1. What does it show?
2. What imaging would you do next?

ANSWERS

1. An obvious swelling of the whole of the right leg and lower abdomen, with obstruction to the right ureter at the level of the pelvic inlet. No bony deposits are seen.
2. A CT of the abdomen.

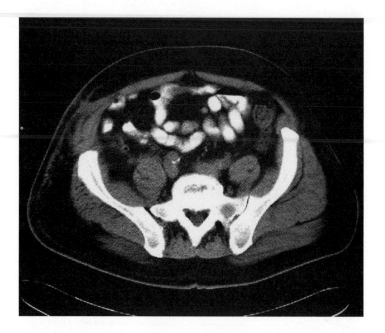

Above is a slice at the level of the pelvic inlet. Interestingly, this shows no gross mass at the level suggested by the bone scan, so presumably there are melanoma deposits surrounding the ureter and iliac vein exerting a sufficient hydrostatic pressure to cause obstruction.

TEACHING POINT

● Although bone scans primarily show the skeleton, remember that the bone agent will also show other abnormalities (see p 32). Melanoma is also well demonstrated on PET imaging, which may show deposits not apparent on CT. Ultrasound with guided biopsy would also be helpful.

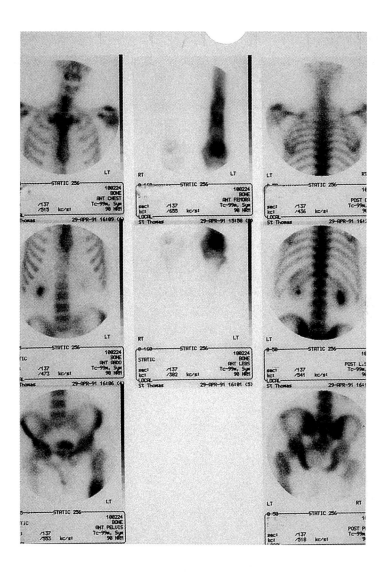

This is a bone scan of an adult patient.

1. What abnormality does it show?

ANSWER

1. Irregularly increased uptake in the left femoral shaft. This is typical of osteomyelitis.

It is also important to compare these findings with X-rays.

TEACHING POINTS

- In the presence of an otherwise normal X-ray, the bone scan is extremely sensitive and specific. It is abnormal before X-rays show periosteal reaction. This is because the bone scan detects the reaction of the bone to early infection whereas the periosteal reaction only occurs when the infection has spread through the bone to the bone surface.
- In the presence of an abnormal X-ray, however, such as in degenerative disease or a Charcot joint, whilst the sensitivity of bone scanning is still high, the specificity is low because the primary abnormality causes increased uptake of tracer in its own right.

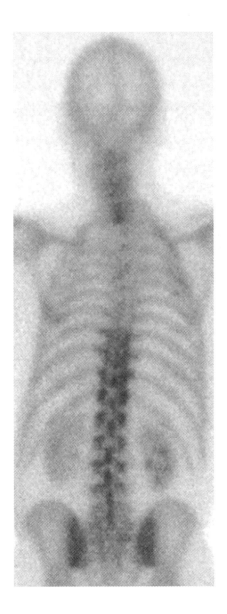

This patient has had treatment for carcinoma of the bronchus.

1. What does this scan show?

ANSWER

1. An obvious long segment of the dorsal spine with generally reduced activity. This is due to the effects of radiotherapy in the past.

Acute radiotherapy changes show hyperaemia. Longer term sequelae of radiotherapy cause fibrosis within the bone and damage the microvascularity of the bone, thus diminishing the blood supply.

TEACHING POINTS

- Uptake within bone is due to blood flow and osteoblastic activity. Where the blood flow is compromised, as here, the uptake will be diminished. Where the blood flow is increased, as in juvenile epiphyses or osteoblastic activity around fractures, the uptake will be increased.
- In this case, the clue is the extent and symmetry of the 'cold' area. Other causes of diminished uptake are extensive rapidly growing tumours and large myeloma deposits.
- Metal prostheses have no blood supply and so are seen as 'cold' photopenic areas.

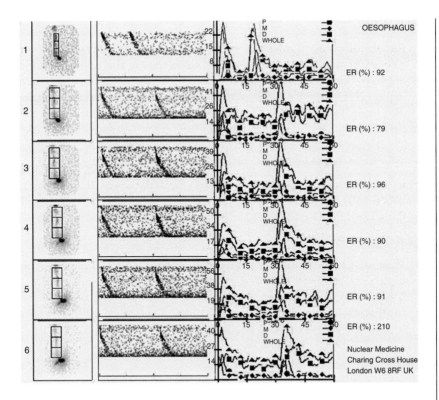

Nuclear Medicine
Charing Cross House
London W6 8RF UK

This patient presented to the gastroenterology department complaining of vomiting after meals. A barium meal and endoscopy were normal.

1. What do these graphs show?
2. How are they done?

ANSWERS

1. Rate of oesophageal clearance of ^{99m}Tc–tin colloid–labelled food.
2. The act of swallowing is repeated six times, giving the six lines on the graph. In this case, the patient only swallowed half the amount, and then whilst being studied, swallowed the rest. This accounts for the two peaks seen in each image and graph. Regions of interest are drawn around the oesophagus, which are then divided into three – upper, middle and lower oesophagus, and time–activity curves are produced. The program gives the emptying rate (ER) as a percentage; 100% is normal.

This study shows normal clearance of tracer, indicating normal oesophageal clearance with no reflux.

TEACHING POINT

- This test can be combined with gastric emptying studies and both are superior to barium studies in providing physiological information about rates of emptying. The transit times depend on the composition of the food given. This needs to be standardized and local normal values established. Transit time for liquid is different.

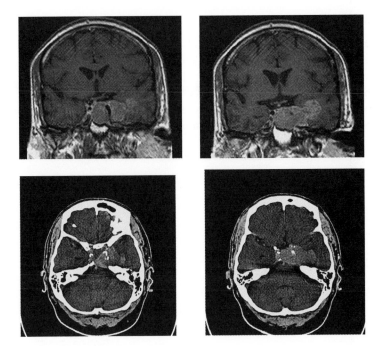

This patient with a known prolactinoma complained of recent onset of headaches and double vision. There had been previous surgery and radio-therapy some years ago. Laboratory tests showed a raised prolactin.

1. What are these investigations?
2. What do they show?
3. What would you do next?

ANSWERS

1. MRI and CT.
2. A very large pituitary tumour extending to the left and encasing the carotid artery (shown as a black flow void on the MRI). The optic chiasm is well above the tumour.
3. An octreotide scan to show whether there are any other foci of somatostatin-secreting tumour within the body.

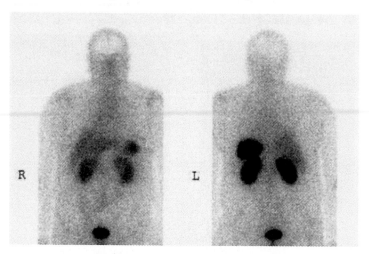

The whole body octreotide scan showed normal distribution in the liver, spleen and renal tract, but no other lesion. SPECT of the head (below), thorax and abdomen was then carried out.

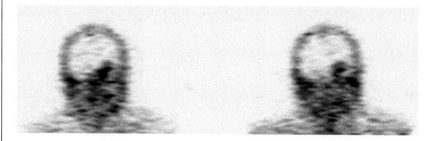

The abnormal uptake in the pituitary region is now clearly seen and matches the MRI images. No abnormal uptake is seen anywhere else in the body on SPECT.

TEACHING POINT

- The value of the octreotide scan is that it shows the tumour to be rich in somatostatin receptors and whether there is one tumour or several. If no further surgery is possible, the tumour might be treatable with either medication, such as cabergoline, or local radiotherapy. In cases with multiple lesions, treatment may be with ^{90}Y-octreotide.

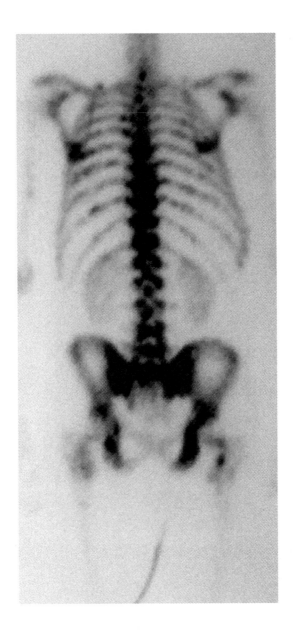

1. What does this bone scan show?
2. What other imaging modality could be used?

ANSWERS

1. Multiple areas of abnormally increased uptake throughout the whole spine, so the statistical likelihood is that of metastatic disease. The activity is so great, the image looks blurred and is almost a 'superscan'. The patient is catheterized, so the likely diagnosis is cancer of the prostate.
2. MRI can also demonstrate deposits.

This MRI below shows the widespread altered marrow signal, typical of deposits.

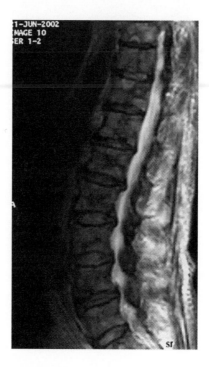

TEACHING POINTS

- MRI is more sensitive than bone scanning in showing deposits and there is no radiation, making it safer and more acceptable under IR(ME)R regulations. However, MRI is not as widely available and the waiting time for imaging may be unacceptably long.
- In a bone scan, uptake is a measure of bony reaction to a metastasis and not the metastasis itself. In general, sclerotic lesions take up tracer because the metastasis causes an attempt by the surrounding bone to repair itself. In lytic osteoclastic lesions, bone scans are not so sensitive and may give false-negative results. This is why bone scans are not used in myeloma.

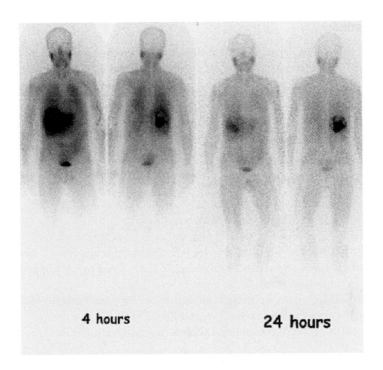

4 hours   24 hours

This is a study performed on a patient with a recent onset of hypertension.

1. What does it show?

ANSWER

1. The ^{123}I-MIBG (metaiodobenzylguanidine) whole body scan shows a large region of increased uptake in the right adrenal region, best shown on the posterior images.

SPECT images may also be obtained. It is important to have a recent CT scan of the abdomen to compare with the MIBG images, as abnormal adrenals may be seen on the CT.

TEACHING POINTS

- MIBG is taken up by the adrenal medulla. Uptake is also seen in the salivary glands and to a lesser extent in the heart.
- Several types of both prescription and non-prescription drugs interfere with MIBG uptake, including tricyclic antidepressants, phenothiazines, amphetamines and nasal decongestants. These need to be stopped for a sufficient period to allow for complete washout.
- MIBG imaging is used in the localization of phaeochromocytomas, para-ganglionomas and, in some cases, carcinoid tumours.
- ^{131}I-MIBG is used therapeutically.

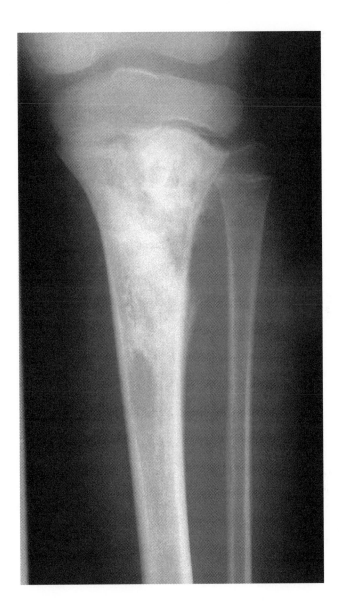

This boy fell over and hurt his knee. As it did not get better, he attended A&E where the above X-ray was obtained.

1. What does this show?
2. What other imaging should be considered?

ANSWERS

1. Irregular sclerosis of the proximal tibia and a raised periosteum that has been breached. The epiphyseal plate is intact. The differential diagnosis is infection or tumour, although tumour is more likely.
2. A bone scan.

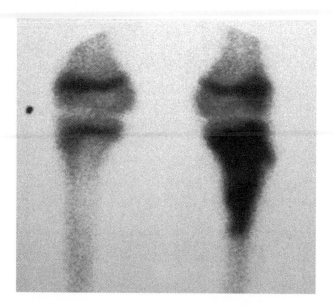

The above bone scan shows the extent of the abnormal bone, compared to the normal leg. Because of the extent, tumour is more likely than infection and this was proved on biopsy. MRI is also conclusive, but a bone scan will show if the disease is multifocal, which influences treatment and prognosis.

TEACHING POINT

- In children, wherever the imaging suggests infection, tumour must also be considered, and vice versa. A biopsy sample should always be sent for microbiology as well as histology/cytology.

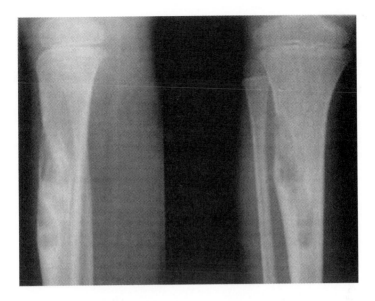

This child hurt his right leg falling.

1. What does the X-ray show?
2. What other tests could be performed?

ANSWERS

1. An area of irregular lucency within the upper tibial metaphysis. The patient is a child – the epiphyses are unfused. There is a sharp zone of transition and well preserved soft tissue planes, suggesting that the lesion is benign. The lesion is often found incidentally, following trauma, resulting in a fracture through the thinned cortex. There is no fracture in this case.

2. Further investigations should include a bone scan.

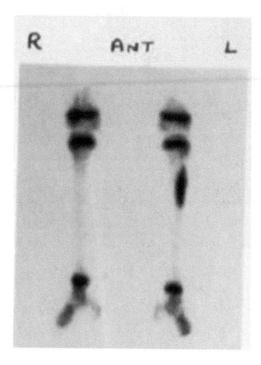

TEACHING POINTS

- The scan shows a well defined area of increased activity matching the bone abnormality. The appearances could be due to fibrous dysplasia, which is metabolically very active, but infection or fracture through the lesion cannot be excluded. Biopsy may well be needed, and remember always to send a specimen for microbiology as well as cytology/histology. This case is an isolated lesion, making malignancy less likely.

- Causes of benign lucent long bone lesions are fibrous dysplasia (either monostotic or polyostotic); non-ossifying fibroma; benign bone cysts; and chronic infection.

- Malignant lesions are either primary (osteosarcoma) or secondaries from neuroblastoma, medulloblastoma, rhabdomyosarcoma, osteosarcoma or teratoma.

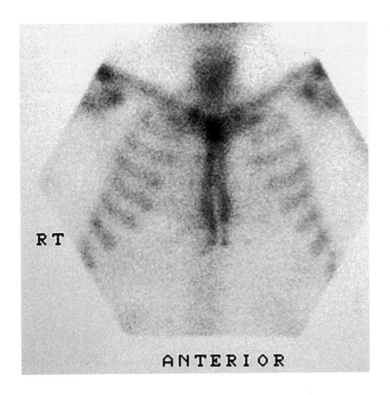

RT

ANTERIOR

This is an anterior view of the thorax from a bone scan series.

1. What does it show?

ANSWER

1. A photon-deficient line clearly seen along the sternum. This represents an unhealed sternotomy performed for cardiac surgery. An unhealed sternum may well be unstable and be a source of pain to the patient.

The sternal sutures and CABG clips can be clearly seen on the chest X-ray.

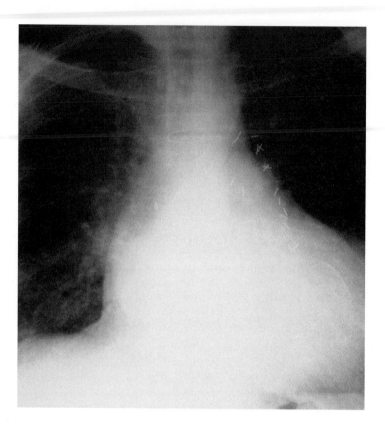

TEACHING POINT

- Photon-deficient areas are due to inadequate blood supply to the bone and are seen where there is non-union of a fracture or where there is a prosthesis. If the surgery was performed within approximately a year of imaging, then there will be increased uptake. Adult bones heal slowly and following a fracture or trauma can take up to 18 months to return to normal.

Regulatory issues

In the UK, the ability to administer radioactive substances is controlled by statute under various Acts of Parliament. Before a suitably qualified doctor is allowed to administer isotopes, he/she must have had suitable training (see p 175). Once trained, he can apply for an appropriate certificate to administer isotopes, and this licence is granted by the Minister of Health who is advised by the Administration of Radioactive Substances Advisory Committee, commonly known as ARSAC.

The certificate applies to an individual medical doctor, to each diagnostic indication and to the premises at which the radionuclide is given, and for diagnostic tests suggests the usual activity that may be given. Under Ionising Radiation (Medical Exposure) Regulations (IR[ME]R) it is the responsibility of the employer to set the diagnostic reference levels (DRLs) for the department but in practice for the majority of tests the ARSAC DRLs are used.

ARSAC issue Notes for Guidance that set out details of the various Acts and how to apply for a certificate. The Notes also list what information is required, how to approach research, special precautions in paediatrics, and of course a complete list of all the radioactive medicinal products commonly used in diagnostic and therapeutic procedures. As well as detailing the radionuclides, this list also sets out the route of administration, the DRL, which is the dose given in MBq, and the effective dose in mSv.

As this list is so comprehensive, the DRL is almost always known in any nuclear medicine procedure, since we work to ARSAC. However, the figures are only guidelines, and in certain cases it may be permissible to exceed the dose, e.g. in grossly obese patients. In these circumstances, the medical physicists in nuclear medicine will be intimately involved in setting the appropriate DRLs.

As well as the ARSAC regulations, there are IR(ME)R 2000 and these relate to the protection of the patient or others receiving a medical exposure. Obviously, these regulations cover all aspects of the use of ionising radiation, not just nuclear medicine.

The general principles of patient protection mean that each exposure must be justified so that the benefit from the test to the patient outweighs the risk of the test, and activities must be kept to the minimum required to obtain a diagnostic image. IR(ME)R sets out employer's responsibilities as well as defining referrers (who are entitled to ask for the investigation), practitioners (whom the employer has designated as taking responsibility for the exposure) and the operator (who carries out the procedure).

All procedure requests must be vetted and justified by the practitioner, who can refuse any request if the form is illegible or incomplete. Obviously, the request will be rejected if it would lead to unacceptable radiation of the patient. Compliance with all of the IR(ME)R regulations for diagnostic, therapeutic and research studies is a complex task, and involves a close co-operation between the imaging staff, both medical and technical, and the medical physics team. It is also the responsibility of the employer to educate all staff so that there is no unnecessary radiation of patients or staff.

Details of all previous imaging investigations must be available for a request to be justified. It is bad medicine to investigate any patient without due regard to the whole picture.

These regulations come under the umbrella of the Heath and Safety regulations and thus any breach of them results in being reported to the General Medical Council.

FURTHER INFORMATION

ARSAC Support Unit
National Radiological Protection Board
Chilton
Didcot, OX11 0RQ
Tel: 01235 832421

The Department of Health web-page relating to ARSAC is on the web at www.advisorybodies.doh.gov.uk/arsac/

IR(ME)R regulations are extremely complex, and you would need to discuss these fully with your medical physicists, but help can also be obtained from the Internet – just enter IR(ME)R on any Internet search engine, and a vast amount of information is available. The Department of Health webpage relating to IR(ME)R can be found at www.doh.gov.uk/assetRoot/04/05/78/38/04057838.pdf

Under the IR(ME)R regulations, inspectors from the Department of Health are authorized to carry out inspections of all imaging departments. Additionally, the British Nuclear Medicine Society (BNMS) audits nuclear medicine departments. Currently, the BNMS audits are voluntary. They are enormously helpful for good practice and preparation for the mandatory IR(ME)R inspections.

After the FRCR or MRCP

DEVELOPMENTS

Nuclear medicine is advancing rapidly and excitingly in the fields of tumour imaging, notably with PET and especially combined PET/CT. There is no doubt that the future of oncological imaging will be with developments in combined PET/CT imaging, especially as modern machines also have an integrated radiotherapy planning program. This means that the patient can be imaged, the tumour identified and located on the CT, and the radio-therapy fields planned, all at one attendance.

Therapy has also seen many recent developments. Advances are being made in adjuncts to recognized therapies, such as the use of lithium to increase the efficiency of ^{131}I therapy in thyrotoxicosis and thyroid cancer, in metastatic palliation therapy with isotopes such as strontium and samarium, and in the treatment of neuroendocrine tumours with yttrium-labelled lanreotide therapy.

TRAINING IN NUCLEAR MEDICINE

Two pathways can be followed to obtain the further training specializing in nuclear medicine, leading to the nuclear medicine CCST. The first, aimed at physicians, takes 4 years and is made up of theory and clinical work based at an accredited centre. As well as diagnostic work, the course also covers laboratory work, PET and therapy with unsealed sources, both for benign and malignant disease. During this training period, the MSc in Nuclear Medicine is usually taken. Currently, this is based at King's College in London, and this degree is usually studied part-time over a 2-year period. The course is modular, with taught components, practical work and a thesis. The overall length of training in nuclear medicine for physicians is such that there is a possibility of working towards an MD. The CCST is awarded at the completion of training, and this allows the acquisition of an Administration of Radioactive Substances Advisory Committee (ARSAC) certificate, both for diagnostic and some therapy work. This course is run under the aegis of the Royal College of Physicians of London.

The second pathway is aimed at post-FRCR radiologists. To acquire an ARSAC certificate, further training beyond the FRCR is needed, and the minimum is to spend Year 5 of the Specialist Registrar programme in Nuclear Medicine. This will allow the radiology registrar to obtain recog-nition in Radionuclide Radiology, but does not lead to a CCST in Nuclear Medicine. It does, of course, count towards the CCST in Radiology. Year 5 work covers all aspects of nuclear medicine imaging with the exception of PET.

For dual accreditation, Year 6 must also be spent in nuclear medicine, and during this year, experience will be gained in in vitro work, PET and therapy.

The post-FRCR Nuclear Medicine training is thus either 1 or 2 years, the 2-year option leading to CCSTs in Radiology and Nuclear Medicine. This course is run under the aegis of the Royal College of Radiologists. The 1-year option, whilst not leading to a CCST, may be attractive to those radiologists who wish to work in a general hospital department where nuclear medicine is available. As about 70% of nuclear medicine as practised in the UK is performed by radiologists, this option is appealing. Those radiologists who wish to work mainly in nuclear medicine in a bigger centre will obviously choose the 2-year option, involving the MSc as described above.

There are currently about 18 accredited posts for further training, and these are open to either post-MRCP physician trainees or post-FRCR radiology trainees. A list of these posts is available on the British Nuclear Medicine Society website (www.bnms.org.uk), but is constantly being enlarged and updated as more training centres get accreditation for training posts in nuclear medicine.

The Royal College of Physicians and the Royal College of Radiologists work together to accredit the training posts whilst separately supervising the two different pathways. The MSc is of course open to all trainees.

CONCLUSION

Nuclear medicine is a very satisfying and rapidly changing method of applying a multi-faceted approach to overall patient care. An additional attraction is the possibility of an acceptable work/life balance.

FURTHER INFORMATION

British Nuclear Medicine Society (www.bnms.org.uk)
Royal College of Physicians, London (www.rcplondon.ac.uk)
Royal College of Radiologists, London (www.rcr.ac.uk)
Society of Nuclear Medicine (www.snm.org)

Further reading

Benard F, Romsa J, Hustinx R. Imaging gliomas with positron emission tomography and single-photon emission computed tomography. *Semin Nucl Med* 2003; 33:148–62.

Cook G, Dutton J. *Exercises in Clinical Nuclear Medicine.* London: Martin Dunitz, 2003.

Ell P, Gambhir S (eds). *Nuclear Medicine in Clinical Diagnosis and Treatment* 3rd edn. Edinburgh: Churchill Livingstone 2004.

Habibian M, Delbeke D, Martin W, Sandler M. *Nuclear Medicine Imaging – a Teaching File.* Philadelphia: Lippincott, Williams and Wilkins, 1999.

Maisey M, Britton K, Gilday D. *Clinical Nuclear Medicine.* London: Hodder, 1991.

Peters AM (ed). *Nuclear Medicine in Radiological Diagnosis.* London: Martin Dunitz, 2003.

Silberstein E, McAfee J, Spasoff A. *Diagnostic Patterns in Nuclear Medicine.* SNM Press, 2000.

Taylor A, Schuster D, Alazraki N. *A Clinician's Guide to Nuclear Medicine.* SNM Press, 2000.

Thrall J, Ziessman H. *Nuclear Medicine: The Requisites,* 2nd edn. St Louis: Mosby, 2000.

There is a large selection of paediatric nuclear medicine images available at www.medical-atlas.org.

An extensive summary of the uses of PET is given by S Gambhir et al in a tabulated summary of the FDG PET literature. (*J Nucl Med* 2001; 42 (Suppl):

Index of cases